Overcoming
the P.I.T.S. of Health

To: Dearest Norma
All the best in
all that you do!
Continue rising
to the top!

Love, Jennifer Denniel

Overcoming the P.I.T.S. of Health

A Guide to Achieving Wholeness
in Every Area of Your Life

Jennifer Desmond RN

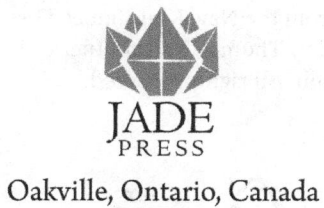

Oakville, Ontario, Canada

Copyright © 2016 Jennifer Desmond

Published by Jade Press, Oakville, Ontario, Canada
www.jadepress.net

All rights reserved. The use of any part of this publication reproduced, transmitted in any form or by any means, electronic, mechanical, recording, or otherwise, or stored in a retrieval system, without prior consent of the publisher, is an infringement of the copyright law. In the case of photocopying or other reprographic copying of the material, a license must be obtained from the Canadian Copyright Licensing Agency (CANCOPY) before proceeding.

Library and Archives Canada Cataloguing in Publication
Desmond, Jennifer, author
    Overcoming the PITS of health : a guide to achieving wholeness in every area of your life / Jennifer Desmond RN.
Issued in print and electronic formats.
ISBN 978-0-9938272-0-4 (pbk.).--ISBN 978-0-9938272-1-1 (kindle).--ISBN 978-0-9938272-2-8 (epub)

    1. Health--Popular works. 2. Stress management--Popular works. 3. Health--Religious aspects--Christianity--Popular works. 4. Well-being. I. Title.
RA776.D47 2016   613   C2014-908053-0
                                           C2014-908054-9

Cover design and text layout:
Simone Gabbay Associates, simonegabbay.com

Printed in Canada

Scripture taken from the New King James Version®.
Copyright ©1982 by Thomas Nelson, Inc.
Used by permission. All rights reserved.

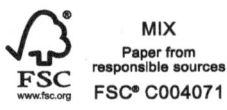

In Appreciation

This book is dedicated to all the mothers, teachers, physicians, nursing mentors, friends, and other professionals who were very important mentors to me at some point and time in my life. I am forever grateful for the professional relationships that helped me find my own PITS.

A special thanks to all the women I met in the community while working as a volunteer nurse and parish nurse. It was in servicing you and addressing your specific personal needs that I was able to identify my own needs and was ultimately led to discover the PITS of Health that lay dormant inside me. This discovery also motivated me to want to equip other professionals who are working in the field of servicing others to invest in their own health to prevent PITS of their own.

I offer my gratitude for all the opportunities I have had to work with other professionals outside of the field of medicine and nursing. I welcome the new friendships that were developed as a result of my writing this book.

I also appreciate all the readers who will make this book their starting point to reclaiming health in their own personal lives. All the best!

Disclaimer of Contents

This book was written to help leadership professionals improve their health by working with the many principles covered within its pages. It was not intended to discriminate against any persons living with a disease or negative condition, but to offer another perspective based on my experience serving others in many situations as a Faith Community Nurse.

The book was not written with the intent to discourage anyone or to refute the assistance of a doctor or any therapies that may be undertaken, but to offer a way to assist the reader through self-empowerment and to manage the outcome by adding the spiritual dimension that may not be widely addressed in society today. The author will not assume liability or responsibility for any outcomes.

The recommendations in this book are based on my experiences and opinions derived from applying many simple forms of therapeutic applications in my work with many individuals. I have also applied many of the concepts to my own health. Others stem from those who have shared their own spiritual practices and behaviors as suggested within the book. The complementary treatment techniques suggested here have also been successful in helping many on their own personal journey to effectively manage their mental and overall physical health.

I would like to make it clear that the term "PITS"[1] is not an established medical term, nor is it known or recognized by other practitioners in the medical and nursing professions. Rather, "PITS" is a term I developed for the purpose of this book and my work with individuals and groups. The term is based on an acronym to help define a condition marked by stress-based, debilitating health challenges that affect professionals and caregivers in many walks of life.

For the diagnosis and treatment of any disease, you are advised to consult a licensed physician.

---

[1] PITS is an acronym for ***P**ersonal **I**ndicators **T**ransforming **S**tress*

Contents

Preface xi

Chapter 1
The Foundation of Health PITS 1

Chapter 2
**What Are the PITS? How Do I
   Discover Them?** 15
   Codes of Ethics for Personal Health,
   Finance, and Relationships 43

Chapter 3
Oh Great, I Have PITS—What Now? ... 51

Chapter 4
No Comparisons 71

Chapter 5
**Getting Out—
   Balancing Health and Life** 93

Chapter 6
Spirituality on Purpose 101

Chapter 7
**How to Develop
 Your Personal Tracker** 125

Chapter 8
Principles 1 – 10 135

Chapter 9
**Reaching Out,
 Setting a New Foundation** 151

Chapter 10
Practice What You Preach 161

Chapter 11
**Perseverance—A Determining Factor
 for Longevity** 167

Chapter 12
Success Indicators 173

About the Author 181

Preface

Just a few years prior to writing this book, I was very successful both in career and in business. That time, in fact, was the most successful time of my life. I had a few minor health issues, but considered myself very healthy overall. I did not even entertain the possibility that these minor health issues would ultimately pose serious threats to my health and well-being. The PITS hit me when I least expected it and eventually stole my health, career, and professional life.

I had gone on sick leave from my job as a surgical nurse after a medical procedure had accelerated the collapse of a very large fibroid that I had carried for many years. I was subsequently prescribed a year-long recovery program that was cut short by a car accident that complicated life and health even more. The accident was debilitating in many ways and its aftereffects and consequences continue to challenge my beliefs, values, and core ideals to this day. Even today, I still feel challenged in my spirituality, my health, and the purpose I thought I had in life. The accident also challenged my livelihood with a total disability diagnosis, right side body pain, and restricted the quality of living in many, many ways. I eventually had to resign my position as a surgical nurse and lay aside a career that I had held so dearly as my most prized possession in life—a job I loved and my invaluable experience as a nurse that gave me the feeling of being a true professional! Facing the prospect of losing a successful career, encountering health issues as a result of a car accident, and experiencing PITS that I had kept dormant inside me, I fell on a slope that unleashed a world I never knew existed—the world of PITS in my own health.

Nevertheless, although I have had to face these PITS and have defeated the majority of them, I still have a long way to go. It is my hope that my personal journey and my experience of serving others stuck in PITS of their own will help you to come to a place of complete introspection and to look within to discover your own destructive PITS. I hope that this book will provide the inspiration and motivation you need to not only identify your own PITS, but also to persevere and dismantle each one as you take control of them in order to have a fruitful and beneficial life. I wish you the very best as you dispel the PITS and move into a time and space propelling you into greater health, happiness, and success in all areas of your life.

This book is written in simple terms and is intended not only for nurses, physicians, engineers, or other professionals and those in leadership positions, but also for lay persons who would like to be equipped with unfailing principles for laying a better foundation for life, finding balance, and ultimately escaping the dangers of the PITS of Health. It is written for everyone whose schedule is anything but peaceful and who would like to harness a quick and easy way to take control of their life and health, especially in today's fast-paced world. I hope you will truly enjoy and find something within this book's pages that will be useful if not meaningful at its best! God Bless you!

Sincerely,

Jennifer Desmond, RN, BScN (c), Parish Nurse

CHAPTER 1

The Foundation of Health PITS

Life has many ways of testing a person's will, either by having nothing happen at all or by having everything happen all at once.

~ Paulo Coelho

Life can be very fulfilling when everything exists in a state of calm—at least in a state of calm that is manageable for us. This calm conveys a false sense of assurance that many of us live in today. Until real tragedy hits our lives or we lose our jobs due to ill health, we may never know how much we take balance, peace, health, and happiness for granted. It is before calamities come upon us or before we feel empty inside that we may be creating PITS in our lives and in health without even consciously knowing.

PITS are developed through our social, mental, emotional, and spiritual values and through our personal beliefs and thoughts about ourselves. Dormant until the opportunity arises for PITS to manifest, many of these PITS stay hidden inside of us. When PITS come alive, they become the very enemy that threatens our ideals; they threaten everything we ever knew. When we have an encounter with the PITS, a slope is created that leads to excessive health challenges both internally and externally. These PITS rob us of the very life we dream of living. The PITS lay a foundation that leads to nowhere except pain, isolation, disease, self-pity, low self-esteem, poor work habits, increased absenteeism, rocky relationships, and very little satisfaction even in the midst of a glorious and highly successful life and career.

When my parents migrated to Canada in the late 1960s, it was an opportune time to start a new life for many families. My grandmother, who was very religious, lived with us, and my sister and I were raised in a strictly disciplined yet highly dysfunctional home. Like most families back then, we had our issues. We were a very large family that included three step siblings and three of our cousins who also lived with us. I had been fondled by my uncle who had stayed with us for a brief time. The camp leader, who was in charge of the Vacation Bible School I attended as a child, also had his piece of the pie. He would kiss me on the lips every time he saw me. At that point in my life, I was a happy-go-lucky child with a lot of issues that many of my family members were not aware of. As I grew into a young woman, by the time I had reached my twenty-first birthday, I had been gang-raped and become homeless and a high school dropout. When I look back at my life now, I wonder how I ever amounted to anything, having had such a dysfunctional life. Why did I not turn out insane and a total nerd, isolated in a box with no future to look forward to? The reason is that each dysfunction takes a new face each time it occurs because we manage to deal with it somehow.

When things are far from perfect, the focus on the difficulty or circumstance we are in becomes blurred and we find ways to cope. We might even rewrite the script of the situation in our minds just so we can stop the hurt, pain, and suffering.

When we meet people who want to become a significant part of our lives, we file the requests away in pockets that bring a degree of comfort, peace, and safety. This is a protection mode that pops up to protect us from repeating what we don't want to face again. In this manner of dealing with our painful or unhappy experiences, some stay lapsed in a space and time and never get filed away, and because they are so painful, we just dare not ruffle the wings of despair again—after all, it happened in the past. These are tricks that our mind plays on us because of our insecurities, former beliefs about ourselves, or even a state of mind based on the foundations we have been living with. This occurs for happy moments, too, especially if we have not experienced a happy moment for a long time. Some happy moments, however, will get sabotaged by other, more powerful and negative experiences, even though they may end in a happy way. Thoughts and feelings left unsolved, whether good or bad or too painful, will stay idle and will lodge themselves in this holding place of our memory, thoughts, and emotions. Eventually, these feelings change our internal environment and start to manifest changes in our body.

There are many scientific studies based on these phenomena. We have read about them in numerous books and articles. It has repeatedly been demonstrated that chemical reactions in the brain change when stress is absorbed by the body on a regular or continuous basis. What we say and do will influence our thinking and our circumstances, which in turn will influence the activity in the brain. Eventually, these stresses will cause a negative chemical reaction and start to manifest themselves through the disease processes. I have read many studies on the topic of how our thoughts and the activities of our mind closely influence each other, and would like to share one here—a study from the Medical Society at Harvard University conducted in December 2011: *http://www.health.harvard.edu/healthbeat/focus-more-to-ease-stress*.

One of the objectives of this book is to explain how the simple intricacies of life have a deep grip on our health, whether or not we are aware of how our conscious and unconscious thoughts and feelings are affecting us. Whatever our professional background is, we all face similar issues, circumstances, and fears. The big difference comes from our coping mechanisms—how focused and in control we are of our thoughts, and ultimately also of who and/or what our driving force is. In her groundbreaking book *Switch On Your Brain: The Key to Peak Happiness, Thinking, and Health*, neuroscientist Caroline Leaf explains how positive thoughts will change the DNA in our body to produce positive or good results. Negative thoughts, on the other hand, will change our DNA to produce the negative aspects we face each day! How grounded are we in our faith, or even how strongly have we conditioned ourselves to be emotionally? But even the most highly equipped individuals—professionals in any walk of life—will at some point fall into difficulty with their health, have fears, and may need a mentor to help them sort through certain issues or to receive some kind of support in circumstances that are too big for them to control. No one is ever excluded from this aspect of life. I believe that at some point in our lives, we all forget the important lessons we have learned about coping, control, and focus, especially at a time of desperation, when we face fears and possibly the threat of death, whether our own or that of a loved one. This applies to people of all ages, all nationalities, and all socioeconomic groups. Oftentimes, we may need to return to a point of reference in order to refocus our thoughts and energies on solving our issues and becoming successful again. It does, however, take more effort when it comes to health and disease, to move past focusing on the negative outcome and to see the positive things that can be gleaned immediately.

The steps to recovery are not always easy, especially when we think we might benefit from following a path that was helpful to another person who underwent a similar metamorphosis. Nor is it always easy to obtain and pay for the services and advice of a professional psychologist or psychiatrist to work through issues of emotional or mental stress. Seeking out these professionals, and even working with tips from grandma's book of wisdom, may still fail to help us. These methods may help a little, but not fully. Our greatest help will come from a source that has nothing to do with any person, skill, or procedure—it will come from a higher source that also lives within each of us and that seems to reveal itself at the point where personal strength is no longer apparent. The only real revelation will come through a small voice or the sudden clarity of direction that you receive in your innermost being, which will lead you to discover yourself in a new and different way. It is when we ignore this deep inner feeling and carry on as usual that things continue to happen behind the scenes that will affect our health and circumstances. The conditions or situations that we face are processed by us based on our interpretations of previous experiences by the brain or through the means of rationalization.

The brain and the mind are two different entities. The brain houses the mind and will control the body, but the mind will control the brain. Our thoughts and experiences are thus often filed away into the deeper realms of our psyche, and we then develop new interpretations, which are, however, still based on old assumptions. Some of our thoughts and emotions are toxic in nature because they are based on these old assumptions and the mind-conditioning and foundations that we started out with. Initially, there may be no noticeable manifestations, but the continued subtle process of filing these thoughts and experiences away or ignoring them may ultimately manifest in emotional despair or physical illness—resulting in the PITS of Health.

You can see by now how easy it may be for us to slip into situations that create a downfall to our health, relationships, and the services that we offer as professionals. Professional service is strictly scrutinized by all. Everyone, including those who appear less fortunate or disadvantaged socially and economically will oftentimes rate services, rate professionals, as well as their experience with certain organizations that provide a service. Servicing others is a vital part of our lives; we encounter it almost daily. It is easy to recognize when we have received unacceptable service that just did not meet our expectations in many ways. The same is true for creating PITS of Health. We are truly affected even by the way we are treated by the people we meet daily. Our thoughts and beliefs move us from one experience to the next, and we react accordingly to each experience, either with pleasure or distaste, prompting chemical reactions that cause our brain to rewire itself to process the thoughts and feelings that flood the body and affect our five senses.

Let's say, for example, that you never took care of yourself properly. You are always skipping meals, fight a lot with your spouse and children, are always in a hurry going to your meaningful job...someone comes in for the service at your place of business. You may mean to treat them differently, but they might have not smiled at you or may have not said a simple word such as thank you and that threatens your self-esteem as you ponder why they reacted to you the way they did. Then, the next person who comes to you gets the brunt of the punishment because you were still trying to sort out the previous client's reaction. Or the opposite occurs where you are trying very hard to be polite and you display a fake smile and pleasant attitude to get through the time that you need to spend with that person because dealing with them and serving them is very stressful for you. In each of these instances, we are caught in a performance that is unhealthy, not only for the person we have served, but mainly for ourselves while we are performing that service. We are left straddled by our emotions, trying to find peace and the meaning of what is occurring and why it is affecting us the way it is. This will especially affect those who are struggling with self-esteem issues. Cognitive dissonance occurs, irrational thinking and maladaptive behavior is introduced at the cellular level, groomed daily through decisions and carried forth into the professional image until it is formally or clinically addressed.

Many of us will rack up points in this category easily because this occurs on a daily basis for many months and even years, until one day we become unfriendly, unhappy, untouched by warmth and love or because it seems to us that the world has not been very fair and we don't know why. Many of these negative emotions do not arise overnight; they are being built up every day, every month, and every year of our lives. As our bodies, through the five senses, send interpretations to the brain, the brain rationalizes these interpretations and will then feed this information to the mind. Through this process, the brain sends a signal to adjust the chemical reactions in our DNA every time this process occurs, and the mind will start to prompt the brain to perform the outcome, whether positive or negative.

Understanding the above concepts could make life so much more meaningful for us. Can you imagine the professional who will live like this from cycle to cycle and will never have known how much freer their life could have been just by changing the way they think? Even if you live with a chronic disease, how much more peace you can have just by changing some small practices, changing the way you look and rationalize things, and elevating your thinking to a place where there is the expectation of healing, a brighter outlook on life, a happier self-awareness, and ten times more success in all areas of life. What

I'm trying to say is, we are creating PITS, whether we are aware of it or not.

Other ways that PITS can be laid as a foundation for our life, health, relationships, and services are through our performance indicators. One dictionary states that a performance indicator "provides quantifiable data about the overall success and effectiveness of a business object." Another refers to performance indicators as "criteria in which to monitor someone or a product/service in how well it is doing." So in health, we must consider the various aspects of living that affect our health performance indicator. Some of these would be our environmental health; physical health; social, intellectual, emotional health; spiritual health; and so on. Health is measured in many scientific ways, as well as in natural ways. Another dictionary describes a health performance indicator as one that is "the principle by which individuals and groups of people learn to behave in a manner conducive to the prevention, maintenance or restoration of health." Why do I mention this? It is mainly through this daily operation that feelings, thoughts, desires, self-inflicted attitudes, emotions, and beliefs—positive or negative, inferior or superficial—are fed to the brain by our body via our senses. We create misconceptions and/or other realities that cloud the real meaning and value we place on our lives and how we view ourselves. These thoughts and attitudes will either serve to manifest the positive and free self we long to have, or set us up for PITS to sabotage our health, emotions, and circumstances and rob us of our future. What we say and do influences our body's reactions to a very large extent and will affect our health and will even give rise to the disease process.

CHAPTER 2

What Are the PITS? How Do I Discover Them?

In Chapter 1, I outlined how PITS affect even the best professional. Whether you grew up with a silver spoon in your mouth or lived in a shelter as a teenager, for many of you, there will be something that was not ideal in your life. We also discussed briefly how our personal performance indicators, along with our health performance indicator, can help us to lay solid foundations for either good or bad—foundations that cause us to be prone to either health or disease. Foundations for PITS can be found in all areas of our lives. There are PITS in our health, service, friendships, relationships, finances, mental health, emotional health, and many more, even in our careers as leaders and professionals. There are PITS even in our most meaningful intentions for ourselves in the way we make and execute decisions, and for others, the way we respond or feel about them. Our foundations have been misconstrued—what we wire into the brain via the body will be reflected in our thoughts, actions, beliefs, and traditions. This process is always transforming and will change our internal and external environments. We will need to start at the very beginning to arrest this cycle and stop the trend leading to nowhere except destruction.

One very profound reason for me in writing this book is that, after I had received the diagnosis of total disability, I first refused to accept it. I also had to come to grips with the foundations that set me up for this diagnosis in the first place—the things I had encountered as a child, as a teenager, and even as a young mother, whether I was mature or not. Not all of us will be privileged to receive the best health education possible. A good understanding of how our body affects the mind is something that, unless it is taught to us, we would not be aware of.

It can only come to us when we arrive at the awareness that there is something much bigger than we are, something that we, and everyone, are part of. This awareness usually comes over time. We must intentionally seek out experiences that further this awareness as we search for meaning in the problems and questions that arise as part of daily living.

In my role as a volunteer nurse in the community, I have found that even the best health professional tends to forget many tools that would equip them to work through their own personal ordeals. They have either lost that knowledge, which happens when we panic, or have never really learned it well enough to be able to draw on it in times of personal need. Some of us are too proud to ever admit that we need help. Others err on the side of caution and admit that they need assistance, and in searching for answers, discover that there is no truth as absolute as that found and based in the words of God.

Our faith always seems to come to the forefront when we are desperate for answers to some pressing issues that we face in life. The bottom line is that a professional is a person, regardless of background, status, or skill and will also face obstacles that hamper their ability to focus clearly. Self-help does not always work on stubborn areas with very deep roots. We obscure our complexities behind the veil of a "professional." The crippling fears we are sometimes facing are also those that are present in clients who deal with the same issues and anxieties and stresses in life as we do.

Another motivation for me in writing this book is that health education is key even to the wise person. Health education is so important to each of us and should be greatly emphasized in our day-to-day living. I will repeat this again: health education is important to each of us, and many times our lives will be a living testimony to others in more ways than one, just by sharing information. Even with the vast number of years of study, courses taken, and health research I have been involved in, I have gained much expertise from many professionals, leaders, and teachers regarding the importance of making sound health decisions daily and sharing this information to benefit our community. As experts, we are not all equipped in the same ways as some of our colleagues, but we all have relevant information that we can share to better the lives of the people around us. Having said this, I was able to write this book based on my own truths as a professional; on the testimonies from others I have worked with; the medical and spiritual breakthroughs that I have experienced, that others have shared with me; and on recent breakthroughs in both the natural and scientific worlds.

In a book written by two nurses for other nurses, *From Silence to Voice: What Nurses Know and Must Communicate to the Public*, the authors, Bernice Buresh and Suzanne Gordon, point out that nurses often do not speak up! Everyone has a voice, can be heard, has something to share, and can make a difference in society. Not many of us, however, will take that first step to share expert knowledge we have gained in practice concerning how to improve one's health, or advocate for healthy living environments within the communities, or take a stand for anything that might challenge our professional image and might make us feel uncomfortable standing alone, even though it could benefit others to a great degree.

As a professional, a nurse, I am also a human being providing a service I felt I was inspired to offer in order to fulfill my destiny as an individual. Through the transition from being able to practice to writing this book, I can now communicate the perils of the PITS and how to avoid them. After an accident I encountered that changed my life completely, I have not yet mastered everything that is written in this book, but at least I have a plan and a clear view of my purpose. I was inspired to find a way to express myself to alert those who are professionals or leaders, who might not be taking care of themselves for various reasons, whether due to heavy work schedules, illness, or other issues, to be extra attentive to their health and well-being. I was losing focus of my dreams as a nurse overall because all I could do for myself at the time was to reflect on the great times my career had served me amidst pain and discomfort and self-pity. I needed to validate that my existence was still relevant, even if I could no longer practice bedside nursing.

I also know that each human experience is worth every bit its weight in gold. At one time, my identity as a primary care nurse who served others was important for me to validate who I was, but I now have a different understanding. No one is above the other, even though we have all been esteemed differently, coming from many different professional and cultural backgrounds. I felt that my destiny as a surgical nurse had shifted, and so, transitioning from clinical nursing, I must now find new ways to utilize my skills and education to benefit others in a more profound way.

Suffice it to say that, in addressing the PITS, I found there is now a large body of research to substantiate the connection between mental health and the disease process. There is also an important correlation between the faith and health factors. Studies have demonstrated that these factors change the internal environment of an individual, bringing about an unexplainable transformation toward better health or ill health. In this book, I have expounded on this material with powerful ideas and proven suggestions.

It has been said many times that health education begins with people and begins at home and offers the opportunity for us to communicate tools for improving one's health and overall fitness for long life. Effective communication requires information that is pertinent and accessible in order to help provide a positive solution for any deeply rooted and extreme situations relating to stress, anxiety, depression, financial issues, marital and emotional problems, and many other physical, mental, and spiritual states that we encounter as individuals. If misleading or misdirected information is passed down to us when we dialogue with others, it can lead to detrimental side effects not only in health, but also in life. While communication is key, it must also be transparent. When we miscommunicate with others, we create situations that are negative and maladaptive. Our understanding is then transferred by the emotional and chemical reactions the body sends to the brain and the brain sends to the mind. Whatever the results of that feeling or experience are, will surface in our minds, and the chain reaction begins. It then affects our ability to reason appropriately, and this will instigate feelings that were buried in our innermost being, resulting in misjudging either ourselves, the person, or the situation. All of this stems from deeply rooted emotions or deeply held beliefs that may have been buried in our mind from the past.

I call these experiences **Side Effects** and **Life Effects**. Most times the *effects* of an experience, regardless of how intense or how simple they appear to be and how we handle them, will create a life effect that we are forced to live with for the rest of our lives. And life effects will create roads that will alter the grooves in the foundation of our thinking life. Once these grooves are established, in the depth of our subconscious, they will continue to build new and unknown PITS that will transform us and our health as we move forward in life.

There are many profound books written by wonderful authors on how to change the course of one's life while facing any situation one may be presently encountering. Many great leaders in our time have displayed phenomenal work through other written materials to outline personal strategies and well-laid-out plans to gain success in areas of health and well-being. Many highly experienced teachers have also outlined unique ways to becoming successful in every area by addressing our spiritual needs in life through rewiring our thinking to see changes, especially in our health. Even for me, working with these concepts has resulted in a tremendous transformation that has brought a degree of peace and stability to my life. Still others have shared their own personal stories of overcoming adversity by writing about them and the concepts they successfully applied to help themselves.

There are also many books and other publications conveying to the public valuable health information involving nutrition and exercise and other inspiring information that covers generally every area of life. A personal testimony, an experience of triumph, or a medical breakthrough is often debuted in the news, but we tend to overlook it because it sounds too farfetched or too good to be true. Whatever the specifics of the story, there will be one theme that runs through them all: the journey might have taken many roads, but in some way, all journeys are ultimately about a step that was taken, an introduction to or renewal of faith, hope that was encountered, and perseverance needed to get through and get out of their crisis—the human journey personalized.

Many will search out truths hidden in their beliefs handed down traditionally, religiously, culturally, or otherwise. Some will develop a desire for a deeper meaning in life, while some, often with the help of others, discover faith. Their journey will take them through many paths to an opportunity to develop a closer walk with Jesus Christ, while others will seek answers only after a crisis of some kind—the death of a loved one, overcoming disease, or facing a medical diagnosis or prognosis. Something inside of us starts to bring forth questions relevant to our awareness of who we are as individuals, our environment, and what this means to us and how it in turn influences our relationship with the rest of the world.

My journey is no different except for the journey itself and that's what makes us all unique in our approach to health and well-being. Our journey is scripted just for us—it is more than just a personal testimony; it is the truth that we live: our personal truth and purpose in life. It becomes a truth that needs to be told and that's worth sharing to better the lives of others. When we do journey to our purpose through this personalized truth and we share this information with others, we impart our truth as a valid means to justify the successful outcome. When we realize that what we experienced was for a greater purpose and transformation of our own human experience, this insight influences and ultimately changes our perspective. I hope this book will help readers who are seeking clarity, better health, and a solution to whatever conflict or turmoil may be clouding their life experiences. It is also my hope that you will find this book an inspiration or a motivation in any area where change is required to transform your life for the better.

Feelings of joy also factor into this equation, because there are times when our journey in joy has plateaued. We find ourselves searching for a new meaning because things appear empty or missing, even when we have everything. What is really needed in the process of building a healthy foundation in erasing the PITS, especially as they relate to health, are happy, peaceful, and joyous times. Peaceful, happy, and joyous times rewire your body, mind, and spirit differently because feelings of contentment and inner peace come from a source far beyond the protons and neutrons that make up the breadth of life as we know it. These feelings are supernatural and will have supernatural yet tangible effects on us, our health, and our lives. This extraordinary force is what has brought science and Bible discoveries together and is now revealing age-old answers to questions that have existed for centuries.

The way we think and respond to any situation can progress or stagnate the process of connecting our natural body and mind to the supernatural pathways of our spiritual self that is meant to keep us whole and disease-free. We endure so much every day and will face so many more highs and lows in health and other areas of life as we progress throughout our life-span, but it is the way we address these issues that is paramount to the outcome.

A person who does not have faith in God and does not follow any religious practices and one who is very dogmatic in their approach can nevertheless go through a similar experience. Even a person without faith will have some sort of a foundational concept that they believe in that is derived from their childhood and upbringing. Whether they feel driven by some higher power or whether they unconsciously believe in God or in Jesus or not, they will still have some form of practice that requires them to solicit help outside of themselves and usually of a higher unseen force, stemming from some sort of faith. When we pray for a miracle to ease the burden or difficulty we are facing, we are admitting to ourselves that we are powerless and need someone or something that has greater power than we do to step in and take over. We hope that our prayer will bring about immediate help, whether we truly believe it will work or not. I now know that prayer connects us with a divine power and supernatural grace that responds to our submissions.

I am part of a social networking site for improving personal health and well-being. On this site, I have met many wonderful individuals with whom I have developed a close bond of friendship. I have even developed a sisterly and brotherly fondness for some of the connections who have similar interests as I do. The main idea of this networking site is to enhance one's well-being through relationships and, I believe, self-awareness of our personal needs. Another objective is to clarify our priorities as they relate to our personal health and take the appropriate action for improving our health. There are all kinds of people from around the world who will post different things about themselves, but these posts always include answers to some type of challenge that we would have received earlier that day by email. The members of this social site receive points for posting comments or smiles and can receive multiple smiles and comments from their various connections daily. It's a great atmosphere and a phenomenal caring online community to be a part of. However, there is an individual on this social networking site who claims to be an atheist. I nevertheless accepted this person's invitation to connect months after reading their daily posts because I thought I could make a difference in their life since I considered myself to be an optimist even in the darkest of the times I personally faced.

One day, I went to my Facebook page and saw that this same connection had made a post about being evicted from their home and that no one would give them a place to live. They had gone from place to place and had nowhere to call home. Both the individual and their partner were out of work. One had applied for unemployment insurance benefits. They were very frustrated by the many failed attempts at getting help and wanted everyone to wish them the best of luck and that the "universe" would grant them their wish of even a one-bedroom apartment. I chuckled, not out of ignorance for this individual, but because such statements still point to the belief in a higher being, even as an atheist. I care what happens to everyone; it comes with a deep concern I have for humanity and the values I hold dearly that led me to become a nurse in the first place. At this point, I also remembered that not too long before that, I had read a post written by the same individual asking everyone to hope and pray for the "universe" to give them a place and an income before they would end up on the streets and die, as it seemed no one cared what might happen to them. Another day, I read a post about what atheists believe, and when the post was made, I immediately saw a reply saying that this individual should address their prayers to God and that He would help them. As I read the post, I realized that the writer who had replied to the post was offering a simple solution by introducing an element of faith so that the individual might become successful in meeting their immediate needs. The writer's suggestion, however, was instantly met with reproach and sinister words, and they were given to understand that they had shown the most horrible disrespect and should be literally cast to death for not respecting the individual's rights and beliefs.

In short and simple terms, even an atheist believes in something. I have read several studies explaining the reasons and demonstrating that even an atheist believes in God unconsciously. Some of these studies are available on the Internet. Our beliefs all stem from our perception of things and their importance or significance to us. In fact, let me address one issue here: I cannot understand how any person, whether rich or poor, cannot believe that the inhabitants of this earth and all its beauty are beyond evolving from apes, which is pathetic thinking to begin with. There is such splendor in nature, and the various places where people live around the world are so uniquely created in different ways that they speak with a quiet beauty that transcends our perception of art and creativity. How can we, in all of our humanity and intelligence, ignore the existence of God and the factors that provide evidence of a higher being that is always in control, never sleeps, and has a vision of wholeness for us?

As a nurse, I have seen families who are facing a diagnosis or surgery and who do not practice any religion or faith of any kind, still pray to God or still mention His name with hope. I have been asked to pray for safe procedures, return of health, healing, and many other fears that individuals were facing while I served at the bedside. A quote I remember seeing from Les Brown states: "Too many of us are not living our dreams because we are living our fears." I thought this quote was so true, even for me, having recently received the diagnosis mentioned earlier in the book. In a moment, so many areas of an individual's life can change. For me, this one moment would prompt me to retire what I believed was my "destiny as a surgical nurse." Another quote by Mark Twain that states, "Nothing so needs reforming as other people's habits," reminds me that we all are influenced by each other in every area of our lives, whether physical, emotional, spiritual, mental, or economical. We are all influenced by a good degree.

So then, what are the PITS? More specifically, what are the PITS of Health? The term was developed from my own definitions and evolved out of my own personal experiences and crises I have faced. I have also met many other professionals whose lives needed clarity, and their health was out in the abyss somewhere. Many of us, over a lifetime, will experience PITS that alter our foundation of health and well-being and cut short our quality of living, just because we did not take the time to properly invest in our own needs, health, or circumstances or left our options to chance. More specifically, the PITS will have influence over an expected outcome, whether personal or of a more universal nature. These things can fall into any category of life. PITS are usually made up of our habits, belief system, experiences, upbringing, education, tradition, value systems, our fight-or-flight responses, and so forth. They can come from stressors, disease, addictions, social phobias, accidents, depression, disabilities, bullying, misconceptions, miscommunications with others, and more. The end results will always affect our health outcomes in some way or another, and these health outcomes will be different for everyone. For instance, since I have had some significant trauma in my life, my foundation will be laid differently in comparison to that of other people who did not experience sexual assault or as much negativity, violence, or dysfunction in their lives as I did.

In Chapter 4, I address the comparison factor and why we must stay away from making comparisons when we have been bruised and beaten by life already. This can be a dangerous practice to engage in. I have, however, received confirmation through dialogue from many professional leaders and education experts, as well as testimonies from others, to validate much of what is stated in this book in respect of comparing ourselves and circumstances to others. We develop a competitive mind that is not necessary if we understand that we are just one person that makes up the whole plan of life and everyone has something to bring to the table that ties us together in our uniqueness and creates balance in the cycle of life. Even in nursing school, the formal study of medicine and the disease process provided many curiosities for me, leading to my own investigations and inquiries into the work of other professionals that addressed the issue of comparison. Some of these have shared their own experiences or ideas on this topic to show how devastating it can be to try to lay a solid foundation for good health in a weak environment.

One of the roles in nursing in which I have had the privilege to serve is that of a Parish Nurse (Faith Community Nurse). Utilizing my knowledge and expertise, I was able to instruct several congregations, communities, and members of organizations in healthy practices and other aspects of profound importance to improving personal well-being. I even attempted to formally train other nurses in this role who served with me. Through this experience, I came to realize that professionals are very predictable when it comes to taking care of themselves. This is especially true when we are facing a personal crisis. We hide our personal fears as we go through the crisis in hopes of maintaining a good professional image without anyone perceiving that we are going through something very personal. We feel much better when we lose ourselves in the service of helping others; we think this noble task will benefit us more and what we are personally facing will just dissipate. But we hurt ourselves in the long run because as leaders, we unconsciously live from standards or a perception that we have set for ourselves—sometimes these standards stem from a pseudo sense of self-accomplishment, whether we think we are living it or not, and our health becomes secondary in order for us to uphold the roles we play in life. Self-denial creates an identity complex that feeds our emotions negatively, which influences the level we view ourselves from, and in our uniqueness, we will display traits in our behavior that are specific to each person. This shapes our interpretation or rationalization of what we are experiencing. This cycle of feeding our identity complex through self-denial affects us internally and externally, and as we have a deeper need to be wanted or to be successful, we send these dysfunctional signals to our brain to create self-satisfaction, while displacing our emotions and health needs into categories, so to speak. This creates ease physically at the time of our personal crisis, but will lead to PITS in the end. All this occurs simultaneously while we are attending to the needs of others or performing our work. Just the very word "professional" implies that we fit some sort of leadership position or role that gives us the ability to supersede any suffering and that this role makes us immune to any personal vulnerability, whether related to health or other aspects of our lives.

Some leaders or professionals tend to treat others as less than they are because they do not possess the same level of education or degree of intelligence as their own personal standards dictate. Through this action, we escape our own feelings of inadequacy as the focus is placed on the person being mistreated. This is wrong, but continues only because much of what we think we know or have is jumbled up into categories that we have established in our gut feelings and in the interpretations we give to a situation. Our perceptions may be negative or positive, but must still be sorted out within ourselves, within our mind, in order to influence how we live our lives. Some professionals have invested time in exploring areas of importance to them and to work through specific areas affecting their health. If they have been on a very long process of self-discovery/self-recovery and experienced some type of personal fulfillment, joy, or happiness, it is often short-lived. Even in the self-discovery process, our happiness and personal fulfillment will be sabotaged by our personal values, level of emotional stability, and or religious beliefs.

As professionals, we also possess weak areas in our foundation that are not apparent to many of us when addressing the issues or problems we face. This happens only because we focus on our own needs superficially since we are often afraid of what we may find to be the truth about ourselves, so we avoid this area all together. If the problem or a situation we overcame was related to going through and fighting a disease, we still don't take the time that is necessary to recuperate because of the pressures of returning to a job or a position, and proper healing is often cut short. Now that it is over and there are no further interests in reliving the fears that left our focus fragmented, we move on from the experience. The process of finding the courage to fight has knocked the wind out of our sails, so there is nothing left to celebrate in the heart of that leader or professional, even if there is a cause for celebration, after they have come through that really terrible thing.

The idea that the experience has passed and it's time to move on will be much more appealing to us than the thought or idea of going through the experience all over again and having to relive the old fears while trying to develop and establish new feelings or a new outlook without diminishing our role as leaders or professionals once again. We hide in the service we provide daily to others as the professionals we are, but only through a superficial lens, and the cycle starts all over again and our foundational thinking remains corrupt, with nothing really improved.

However, it takes an exceptional leader to have discovered themselves through a higher revelation of self or through a deeper foundational focus that meaningfully explains their existence on this planet. It creates an eye opener to the fellowship that is necessary in a union with God to avoid the destructive ways to live, and as a means to increase faith in God and therefore, in return, to experience the principles of God. These principles include practical steps to achieving success, elevation in knowledge about all things, achieving the desires of the heart, perfect health and wellness, loving service we need to give to others, and a vibrant unique vision for life. This acknowledgment, when realized, is less burdensome to our health and to our body, mind, and spiritual needs. It creates a knowledge or perception of wholeness that leads you away from the PITS of Health and yes, it can be done, even if you are ridden with physical pain, as I often am.

PITS, what is it, then? Please permit me to share this discovery with you. You might have heard another version of it someplace else.

What Are the PITS? How Do I Discover Them?

> **The acronym P.I.T.S. stands for:**
> **P**ersonal **I**ndicators **T**ransforming **S**tress
> – PITS in a person's life

Here it is again:

- **P** = Personal
- **I** = Indicators
- **T** = Transforming
- **S** = Stress

PITS can affect all of the things and conditions previously mentioned and can also include your personal indicators to nutrition, obesity, exercise, social outlets, family, sleep, meditation, career, personal and physical balance, and many, many more. It can cause a great career to crash and a successful journey to come to an abrupt end. By now you may be able to recognize some of your own PITS that will have caused a disintegration of some kind in your life.

To address these PITS does take some technique. Many of us would deny our conditions or circumstances, even if they were presented with evidence. So the first step in understanding or recognizing these PITS is to acknowledge them. In order to be able to work through the ten steps outlined in this book, *you* must get honest with *yourself*. To be able to overcome your position, no matter where you are presently with your health, marriage, career, finances, or other—as a leader or lay person, you must get focus.

Setting aside time in order for a deep recognition to occur can be quite a self-discovery, but it is important. We do not need a degree or a position of leadership to come to grips with what is wrong, broken, or needs to be arrested in our lives, especially in our own health, in order to gain better ground to well-being and balance. We have what it takes inside of us to make any change we are seeking, that might be necessary and includes healing from any disease that was created by past experiences or dormant PITS, engraved in our thinking and our foundational plan for wellness.

The reason I used the word "arrest" in the preceding paragraph is that sometimes there are different degrees of needs or experiences that are so destructive that they continue to eat away at us internally, and these are usually rooted very deeply inside of us because they were probably deposited there a long time ago. Eradicating these PITS will require more than just simple efforts to dislodge them; it may stir up fears of doing anything that might help us to let go and get help. A Spanish Proverb states, "Habits are at first cobwebs, then cables," and the same is true for dislodging a painful experience, a terrible diagnosis, changing health habits, or anything else for that matter.

For many of us in leadership positions or roles, the organization we work for has stipulated a certain code of ethics that is in line with their expectations. If you are not sure of your organization's code of ethics, it would be quite an eye opener to examine it. In nursing, we are governed by the codes of ethics pertaining to our practice that keeps our nursing standards unified under the agreement stipulated by the College of Nurses in order to be accountable while safely practicing nursing. The same is true for us in starting to recognize what is necessary for us in terms of change. If we should develop a certain "code of ethics" for our personal health or circumstance, it will lead us to recognize the drastic changes necessary for our lives and offer a starting point for recognizing areas we are accountable for. It will help to create a tool for us to work with in order to discover avenues that allow us to be ready to address our health priorities or most pressing personal inadequacies or other apparent needs in a methodical fashion.

You could purchase a small exercise book to journal your ideas or concerns as you continue reading this book and to address your needs through the exercises found in several chapters. Please name your journal to make it personal to you, for example, *Jennifer's PITS of Health* (A Personal Self-Development Journal). On page 1, state your own personal ethical reasons for going through and completing this plan to changing any PITS that were dormant or any other PITS for that matter. You can start with simple mission statements such as these: "I am responsible for my personal health, which includes eating, sleeping, and meditation time." "I am responsible for sharing health information with loved ones for better health." "I am responsible for understanding what makes me very angry, stressed out, and how I can incorporate the necessary changes into my life." These are just ideas that I am suggesting, but you could tailor these statements to your own needs and write them in your own words to make them meaningful for you. This is a good place to start as it will help to direct your focus to the tasks ahead.

Code of Ethics for Personal Health

1. _____
2. _____
3. _____

Code of Ethics for Personal Finances

1. _____
2. _____
3. _____

Code of Ethics for Personal Relationships

1. _____
2. _____
3. _____

Here are some suggestions for creating your own Codes of Ethics. Make a list for each individual aspect that is important to you as a professional, a leader, or just someone who is seeking new meaning in their life. No need to limit yourself during this exercise. You can make these lists as long or as short as you wish, but it's important to list ONLY the important areas of your life for which you are seeking changes. Focus!

Another way to help you discover your own personal code of ethics around the PITS in your life is this: you can write out the acronym for PITS and make a list in each section to help bring more clarity to your needs. As you start to write, you will discover other areas or needs to address.

Some Examples of PITS

Personal – Your past history: emotional expressions, personality traits such as a perfectionist or procrastinator; feelings of depression; financial issues or other personal struggles; health response to a diagnosis or sickness of some kind; my marriage has ended because I was working long hours and was never home; everything irritates me; why am I always feeling lonely when I have everything? I have become isolated socially, etc.

Indicators – You might have to take a couple of days to sort out this category for you. Habits, beliefs, and all other value systems would appear in this; experiences can also fit into this category, as well as others; etc.

Transforming – What causes you to interpret things a certain way, dysfunctional attitudes, behaviors; what will take your stress and make it transform? Is it your beliefs, habits, reactions, perceptions, lack of self-esteem, personal insecurities, cultural traditions, delusions of grandeur, etc., that would have encouraged the PITS to develop?

Stress – There should be plenty to fill this category if you are totally honest and transparent with yourself; you can list stressors or situations leading to stressors, irritants, any inability to handle certain circumstances emotionally, any known habits, etc.

> ***A Personal Note:*** *Don't be alarmed if each category seems to be repeated in the other. If you are truly honest with yourself, your responses will be intertwined. Much of what we believe, feel, think, act, and so forth is interrelated, and we usually will make the decisions for ourselves that best suit ourselves without consciously thinking that we desire the highest achievable outcome in all things. This is the whole person in action. All these parts blend into one—one person: you, the leader and professional!*

As previously mentioned, please be aware that some major feelings, words we speak, our interpretation of life, personal beliefs, and more might be present in many of these categories, and that is how it should be. The PITS are intertwined in all areas of life. This is due to the fact that you are a whole person. When you visit the doctor and are being treated for anything, sometimes the physician will address only issues, systems, or symptoms pertaining to your complaint. It may seem as if he or she were only looking at one area of your health, and this might be the case in medicine. But you are a whole person and everything about you, from head to toe, provides a whole picture, even though it might be addressed in part. We are made up of body, mind, and spirit and therefore these cannot be separated. Medical professionals will understand this more than any other professional groups, obviously due to the scientific evidence available to them, their practical experience, as well as many years of studies revealing facts about our physical structure.

It is vitally important to do the Code of Ethics exercise first before pursuing the next exercise of identifying your PITS. You will also almost immediately notice that the codes do not match up with the PITS. Eventually, the PITS will disintegrate the codes, and this usually will shine through in your health. The negative aspects of health will chip away at the positive aspects of health. Regardless of the PITS on your list, you will see the reflection in your codes and vice versa. Much of what you have written will match up, and there will be areas where there may be information gaps that can reveal other areas you may have overlooked that are necessary to confront if you are to be successful going forward.

The remaining chapters of this book will discuss other topics in an in-depth manner, using a step-by-step process to help you to filter through your feelings and devise a plan to assist you to identify your PITS in order to make the transition to becoming the leader or professional you truly desire to become. Arresting these habits, destructive thinking, and ideals that will be detrimental to your health in the long run, takes effort and putting in place steps to discontinuing these pitfalls will be equally important.

Another way to identifying PITS in health is this: in your Personal Self-Development Journal, list the following, side by side, on the same page or divide the page in half. On one side of the page or half of the page, label the column *Life Effects* and on the other side or half label it *Side Effects*. This makes it easy to compare your information. Please list the experiences, especially those affecting health, relationships, etc., in the *Side Effects* column. *Side Effects* can also be identified through the avenue we took to solve problems, the choices we make when under distress, and the steps we took to get to the final destination of acceptance of the outcome. These are to be listed in the *Side Effects* column. List what happened—the end results—what you have lived with or are living with as the final outcome, in the *Life Effects* column.

It is important to focus here and narrow your list down to major events, experiences, or turning points in your life that have made an impact on how you view life in general now. Other examples can be a death or a birth—something very significant. Highlight these two headings, *Life Effects*, *Side Effects,* with your favorite color to signify acceptance or undertaking a new contract with yourself. We will discuss this further in the next few chapters, but for now, focus on the important times you can remember that you didn't want to remember, when "Life" kicked you down, you thought you would never get back up, or when you were down and "Life" gave you a hand and picked you up!

CHAPTER 3

Oh Great, I Have PITS—What Now?

Please relax! You will be fine! That is, provided you are seeking transparency and long-lasting change and want to arrest and disburse the things harming your health that can also steal your career, joy, relationships, finances, marriage, and more. I hope that this book will help you to address the concerns that are invading your peace, tranquility, and ability to live the fulfilled life you were created for.

Reviewing Before Proceeding

So far, you have been writing in your personal journals and working on the exercises in order to make a difference in your role as a *healthy* individual. But sometimes you may have been in denial or unable for other reasons to record your true emotions and deep-rooted convictions so that you could face the PITS of Health successfully.

Let's take a moment to review what you have learned so far in identifying your own personal triggers to developing PITS and to somehow identify how strong your original foundation to health really is. It will also be helpful to review this again at least two more times while reading this chapter to be able to identify any areas you may have missed that need to be included. Also, in order to proceed and have great success, it is imperative that you add any information you may have omitted that was just too painful to face at the time of doing the exercise. By facing these issues now, you can start erasing them from your mind bank or taking back the power they once exercised over you through the limitations of thinking.

For example, in Chapter 1, I stated that by the time I was in my early adulthood, I had been gang-raped, and it had caused a significant health crisis in my life leading up to major surgery. This experience was very painful, and even now, having to remember details of the incident, I still feel a discomfort, even though I have come to grips with the experience and accept that it is now part of the foundation of who I am. I also realize that this dreadful incident did not define who I have become.

Many people who have come and gone in my life never knew that I was gang-raped as a young girl. They never suspected anything simply because I never shared the experience with them or acted in any way that would lead them to suspect that this horrible event took place in my life. Oftentimes handsome men and beautiful women have said to me, "But you are so beautiful and have it all together...I wish I could be like you." I have learned to never wish to be like someone else because one never knows what hell they have endured or are still trying to escape from. Every person has a story to tell—everyone! Yours is equally and vitally important!

In my dating experiences, however, many wise and experienced men have sensed that something negative had happened to me. I was cautious in my actions and sexually reserved. In this regard, even though I did not convey such emotions directly to the men I dated, they were still obvious to some in intimate situations that prompted certain memories to arise. I gave this example because something similar occurs with buried emotions and experiences. We may not fully remember all the details when we have flashbacks of a buried experience or are superficially engaged in dialogue, but deep inside ourselves, in the very depths of our body, at the level of cellular activity, we will remember to some degree. This occurs because the brain connects these memories with similar feelings or experiences as they arise. We also have the natural ability to remember in order to start the process of change, but it takes *focus*! The same is true for recognizing a fear, a hurtful situation, or a change that must be made that no one else can do for you! We must boldly say to ourselves that enough is enough, face the PITS honestly, and succeed in all areas to live happier and healthier lives!

And yes, I know it is not as easy as it is made out to be, but I guarantee you that with one step, you have already changed the course of any PITS or that decision to be made for the better or the worst. Unfortunately, once we recognize the PITS could represent the worst areas of life, and we must once again face these circumstances, we run for the hills—never solving the problem, and this begins a cycle that keeps going until we crash in health, in a relationship, with our finances, through an accident, a diagnosis, or other!

There are many issues we can put on our lists. There are also many books addressing these issues directly. But I am hoping that the words on the pages of this book will be the voice of encouragement to stimulate change for the better, courage to face every area with confidence, regained power to control what happens next, renewal of your thinking and motivation to persevere for those who will read and apply the simple principles or techniques presented. I hope you will use the exercises to confront your deepest fears—fears and secrets you have kept to yourself until now, and other negative experiences that you have not faced openly, the buried dreams, relationship issues, a loved one you have not forgiven. All of these emotions or feelings, whatever we label them, can dissolve. We don't want them added to our lives to create PITS in mind, body, and spirit, but it will take some work for them to be dissolved out of our life

It is never too late for anything in life. It is never too late to change. It is never too late to develop a healthy or holistic lifestyle for all areas of our mind, body, and spirit. We let society dictate to us when, where, and how we should do everything in life—when we should be truly listening to our own inner guidance. Oftentimes when we get a glimpse of the real self and the real issues for what they are in our life, we run away. We run away by avoiding the situation, mentally shutting ourselves off, avoiding any thoughts or desire for thinking toward any part of it or even being reluctant to examine where we could have made a difference. If we take the time to examine ourselves with honesty and true transparency, we will see that there is a much higher source of power present in our lives that makes these actions of ours irrefutable.

If we still refuse to face the issues, especially the ones that influence our mind and thinking, they seep into our physical foundation, which is our body, and manifest from there. Many people steadfastly deny the existence of God, who is in control of us and our being to some extent because He gave us the ability to exercise free will. God's vision for us is wholeness. This is not a statement based on religious beliefs, but on evidence that the supernatural world does exist and it also influences us as a natural or physical, emotional, and spiritual being. This occurs whether we want to be part of this process or not. It is a truth that has been evident since the beginning of time.

The supernatural source of power can suddenly become the main focal point to all of our answers—or problems. It can help us develop strength and courage or strengthen others who are weak in body, mind, and spirit who may believe that God is punishing them and will not help them. These individuals have much in common and may have no spiritual foundation or have lost their faith for some reason or another or have not fully learned who God really is and why He loves us so much and can never punish us through disease, mental issues, or even lack. Many others don't have the spirit to fight for balance because PITS are overpowering their lives due to a lack of understanding of themselves and what they want out of life. They have fought for a very long time, spending much of their physical and emotional selves just trying to stay afloat with all the negative experiences they have had. My question to you at this point, before you proceed further into the book is, what about *you*? How do you want to proceed in your self-development, especially for this year? What about your career choices, your business venture, your family relationships—but mainly for yourself?

I know I got ahead of myself here and mentioned several things.

At least at this point, some more personal reflection will clear the mind's eye and increase focus on how to handle the current PITS that we *have* identified for ourselves. Everything else will fall into place shortly.

So how do we utilize what we now understand about ourselves? What do we do with the PITS to Health that we identified and that are weakening our foundation as an individual? In other words—what now?

On a new page in your Personal Development Journal, write "Dysfunctional Me." That is correct: Dysfunctional Me. Please underline this title with a color you like least for this section of the exercise. Highlighting your dysfunctional list takes the fear out of the unknown areas you once ignored in this category, maybe because of being afraid of any consequences that might arise, from confrontation to any inadequacies stemming from a dysfunction you may have been exposed to while growing up or that you gained as an adult due to your perceptions, actions, or responses. It makes a bold statement to the conscious and unconscious side of your existence that you are ready to face these issues head on with this second step of acknowledgment, even though you don't like it or it will make you feel very uncomfortable.

....

Under the heading, make a subheading.
Please see my example below.

Dysfunctional Me

How have I been functioning in the dysfunction?

....

Now for every Life Effect, there will be a Side Effect. Every Side Effect will involve some sort of *dysfunctional* thinking. List every thought you can think of that would have been positive in handling a terrible situation, a bad circumstance, a happy or unhappy experience, or just a wonderful happy memory overall. Oops, did I say "wonderful happy memory overall"? Yes, indeed! I have found that clients who came to consult me because of some negative issue they were facing would sometimes begin by talking about the very pleasant memories they last stored in their minds regarding the negative situation to be discussed. But upon reviewing what they were telling me, it became apparent that the negative situations in these people's lives were often created by underlying issues that expressed in dysfunctional ways of thinking or could be traced back to negative experiences.

It's important to also clarify that this is not always the case—positive and happy memories that are stored in our mind and heart can come strictly from happy occasions and not always from the pleasant outcome of a very bad thing. Please permit me to state this again. Sometimes the very pleasant memories we store are actually gleamed and stem from a dysfunctional way of thinking or from negative experiences with good outcomes. It's important to also clarify that this is not always the case—positive and happy memories that are stored in our mind and heart can come strictly from happy occasions and not always from the pleasant outcome of a very bad thing. It's almost like having a beautiful picture hanging on the wall that fell, breaking the frame, but the picture was safe and remained beautifully intact, so you just hung it back up on the wall anyway. Likewise, we can frame positive and happy moments into the PITS and foundations of our life, in spite of dysfunction.

Why make a whole exercise solely based on dysfunction? The reason is that sometimes, if we reflect long enough on something that we experienced in a positive way, it will yield wonderful memories. It will also show how it was actually associated with a negative thing, experience, or feeling, just to get to the positive and wonderful end results. There might be some slight disappointment arising that might try to place a shadow on the great moment, but most times we will fight to make sure the outcome remains the same—positive, at least in our mind. It will be of benefit to us in some way, so the fight becomes more real the more we have to fight. This may seem applicable only in the case of an athlete who will work hard for a medal and at the end will have a story of victory despite all the challenges they faced that were tempting them to give up to despair. However, it is also true for many of us in the experiences we have already come through. But for some individuals, the experiences are too deep and painful to desire or motivate the deep need to want to change, or to work toward that medal, reward, peace of mind, healing in the body, a balanced life—whatever it may be. Why do we not think this can also pertain to us? We don't see ourselves and circumstances with the same value as we do our heroes, favorite athletes, or a person we greatly admire or who we think may have it all together—we don't view ourselves as equally important.

I remember one day visiting a family member who found themselves in a really bad predicament. They had just come out of relationship with a person who had promised a better year ahead for both of them. Some of us are only too familiar with the story where you get promised the world. I also experienced this several times in my life. You do, however, have to give up some things. This individual had found themselves in a very small room with their belongings, out of money, unable to pay the rent, cell phone about to be cut off, and had no food. They had given up even their job for the promise of a "better life," because they were going to be moving to another province.

When I saw this individual, I could see they were distraught, searching within for the whys, for "how come these things always happen to me?" and for "I shouldn't have." I noticed there was a plaque on the wall that stated, "Faith is the substance of things hoped for, the evidence of things not seen." I asked what they were truly hoping for in life and why that plaque was on the wall. At one point, they wanted to pray for me, but I quickly responded, pointing out that many of us are always quick to pray for others and claim God's promises for others and never for ourselves. I said that they needed to pray for themselves, their faith, and for the things they were hoping for—to remove the evidence of things they were seeing because at present it didn't seem like life was bringing forth fruit in their affairs and for the things they really wanted to see happening. This is true for many of us. We have the knowledge of what we need, but would rather give that power to someone else to decide for us what we want. We also will pray for the blessings of others and somehow feel we ourselves don't deserve these blessings. We need to love and do these wonderful things for others, but is it vitally and equally healthy and important to do them for ourselves, too. We need this affirming of self, especially when our own lives are falling apart and we need clarity to regain our emotional balance! We surely need to come to a place where we can get focused on our own needs and have them met, and this is not being selfish! Why can't we accept and know that we also have access to these higher principles from God that are available to others and that they can revolutionize our lives as well—to know that we are deserving of balance and great change in all aspects of our lives, too?

Remember, as a leader or professional, you are networking daily through service or other means and will come in contact with people in many ways, shapes and forms, so to speak; how you consciously or unconsciously react may not be important to you, but life is a cycle, and we tend to either feed the positive things or the negative things in the people we meet on a daily basis. This is the ultimate cycle of life, and as much as we feed the emotions of others, we are at the same time fueling our own emotions as well. Even if you are locked up in a room somewhere at some point and time, you will come in contact with another human being and will experience that person on some level while still hiding a part of yourself, or you can die from hopelessness, loneliness, and lack of love in your life.

Why is it that we can see a person, never speak with them, but remember them or something in the way they appeared or did or did not do, or something that will leave an imprint in our minds and that we store away in that image? Well, the same stands true for what is important to us. We have emotional imprints with which we daily infuse ourselves as well as others whom we meet every day—imprints that then get stored away in the cellular memories of being. This happens whether we are aware of it or not. What kinds of imprints are we aware of that we do need to address, remove, or simply delete deliberately for ourselves today that have stuck to our foundational thinking, emotions, and values that are affecting our health?

Another thing is that really focusing and spending time to recognize our dysfunctional attitudes, beliefs, ideas, notions, or whatever we call them will be a great start to handling our PITS and to transforming the platform for the foundation in our thinking that alters our health and well-being positively for years to come.

On another page in your journal, list the headings Life Effects, Side Effects, and Dysfunctions. On this page, note any common themes or reoccurrences from the previous exercise in identifying your dysfunctions. This is sometimes very clear to identify. Don't be alarmed if your Side Effects list resembles your Dysfunctional list. After identifying the common themes of words, thoughts, etc., in your Dysfunctional list, revisit your page on identifying the PITS. Then see if any of those themes were placed in any of these categories as well. Please make a fresh list to include this new addition to the PITS! We want to make sure we haven't missed any areas of vital importance.

Please see examples below:

P -   (what dysfunctions appeared as a personal acknowledgment)

I -   (what indicators or actions now appear as a dysfunction)

T -   (how did dysfunctional transformation occur in my circumstance)

S -   (why do I allow experiences to feed the dysfunctional side of my emotions)

Let's now examine the dictionary meaning of "dysfunction." The Collins English Dictionary & Thesaurus, 21st Century Edition,[2] standard version, defines the term as:

1. *any disturbance or abnormality in the function of an organ or part;*

2. *(esp. of a family) failure to show the characteristics or fulfill the purposes held as normal or beneficial.*

---

[2] ISBN-0-00-472502-6 standard

Here come the *big* questions of the day, after looking at your lists, especially the Life Effects and Side Effects lists:

1. How do you feel about the meaning of dysfunction and how has it influenced your decisions in every area of your life right up until now?
2. Did you expect what you now see about yourself?
3. Does the information about you reflect who you currently see yourself to be?
4. On a scale from 1 to 10, how deep is the dysfunctional level in your foundation?

A positive reflection out of all of this negativity is that once you have accepted your own flaws, and worked through them, no one else can use them against you. Isn't this great news? It sure is—that is the most freeing statement that has ever been written, and I have fully embraced it. In our own microcosm, we can change how we look at the world and our personal experiences by just pausing and becoming aware of our knowingness, power, and need for self-love and forgiveness for our shortcomings. Some people get lost in the simple fact of just trying to find themselves, their own values, and their own truth. It could become burdensome, as it could mean adding to an already busy schedule or create a challenge we are not ready for. It could become a mountain too tall to climb, yet we expect positive results in every way possible. Whatever your value system is interpreted to be, it will be the measure and sum of the types of risks you are willing to take. It will be dependent on how far you are willing to advance the breadth of your actions to any area of your life that is being challenged, in order to receive the benefits and freedom from any limitations holding you back and for the accomplishment you will gain. In many cases, traditional medicine does *not* cure disease or dis-ease. It puts just a masking over the symptoms, but will not cure them. The same stands true for change, gaining personal power, and perseverance. We must fight for what we believe and stick with it to see any kind of results. Every one of us, if we are to be successful in laying new and strong foundations to our health and well-being, must have room to improve each section in our mental makeup and overall expectations of life, not just to put a mask around our issues and cope with the resulting potential chaos, confusion, or ill health.

The truth of the matter is, when you change the way you look at your PITS or just even at the stressors and the general things that steal your joy, the stressor you previously saw now changes. Some of the power has been withdrawn just from facing or looking at the issue more intensely. The more you look at it, the less power it has. Our perception starts to transform the way we think of the issue or how it would affect us; we roll it over in our minds and each time it becomes more diluted until our perception has elevated itself over the thoughts previously held and we appear to be on top of it and it has no effect on us anymore. What has changed? The high standards that once kept these negatives as top priority in our life have now lost their overall power to prevail. The opportunity to develop a new perspective, to strengthen the decision-making process and the ability to renew our mind or thinking now becomes available to us. It is a personal choice to rewire our mind. Not everyone will recognize this at times of reflection, but all of us will have somehow gone through this process. It is what helps us to grow mentally and spiritually and to assist us in changing our mindset, our internal and external worlds or environments.

Here is where your Code of Ethics for your personal health can now be rewritten in a positive light and become paramount in helping you to move forward in all areas of your life with a strong and more powerful conviction and assurance and ability to start the process of reshaping your foundations in the right direction.

CHAPTER 4

No Comparisons

Then God said, "Let Us make man in Our image, according to Our likeness; let them have dominion over the fish of the sea, over the birds of the air, and over the cattle, over all the earth and over every creeping thing that creeps on the earth." So God created man in His own image; in the image of God He created him; male and female He created them.

Genesis 1: 26-27 NKJV

The biggest mistakes we make as human beings are to compare ourselves to others. We compare our physical appearances, our wealth, our education; anything and everything we dare to compare will at some point in time become a reference of ourselves through a comparison to others or to something outside ourselves. I have never understood why we do that. We don't compare ourselves to a chicken or an ox, but this is not necessarily true, either. We do sometimes use expressions such as "strong as an ox" or "humble as a lamb." But why do we do this? Is it because unconsciously we are missing something within ourselves when we engage in any type of comparison? Comparing ourselves to others demonstrates an inadequacy that we have kept buried internally that exposes itself every time we compare ourselves to others. How many of us will compare ourselves to an angel, a prince, someone of high stature, or even a well-known princess? We see television stars comparing themselves to each other in terms of skills, ability, and even beauty. But how many of us will take a stance and say that they are not comparable to anything that currently exists in this world and accept their uniqueness, flaws, and everything in between? To make such a statement with firm conviction, you would have to be very confident in who you are. Yet even the most confident person will feel inferior at the first sign of someone else who might appear even slightly higher in stature or intelligence than they see in themselves.

In the Bible—the book of instruction or what I term the Book of Life—it is written that we were created in the image of God. So what is this image that the good book is speaking of that we were created in? We were created to be perfect in appearance, in ability, skills, every physical area of our life, in our mental capacity, spiritually, and in many more facets of life we would never even consider. Yet, it is easy for us to think, act, and see ourselves as being far from perfect and full of flaws that can't be corrected. Did we walk away from this perfection we were created for in life? Or do we ever come to realize how perfect we really are regardless of our lives? These are serious questions we should be considering. You see, this is where the rubber will oftentimes meet the road again. You might reason that if we are created so perfectly, then why do bad things happen to us? Why are you even reading this book? Can you really change how things continue to happen to you? The answer is yes, yes, and yes! People tend to equate the Bible and perfect living with a religious plight that not many of us can relate to, yet if we truly take the time to understand what the Bible is saying to us, it will instantly change everything about us and everything we thought we knew about ourselves. Before you close the book and be done with it, please let me explain. Religion focuses on the law of right and wrong and leads us to steps that will judge our every action as good, bad, or indifferent. It causes us to compare ourselves to others and also to things instead of focusing on the truths about who we really are and why we were created and why we have been blessed to experience this life. But a true understanding of the man of the Christian religion, Jesus Christ, changes everything. Yes, there is a BIG difference in what I have just written and what is generally believed about Him, the Bible, and how we must live.

At one point in time, before I regained power in all areas of my life, I struggled with this very thought—that one man can make a difference in many lives, changing them for the better if we but come to know him. This man is Jesus—God's only son. God found that the evil in the world was at an all-time high and was grieving over it. He was willing to send His son to a world that would hate Him and kill Him for teaching us a better way to live and not just live from our limited understanding of the world around us, but embrace a higher perspective of life, health, healing from any type of sickness, and have the ability to live happy, fulfilled lives. Wouldn't you want a better way to live if it were available to you? Yet many rejected what Jesus was showing us—ways and values higher than we can see with our physical eyes—and they killed Him. Jesus showed us that there was more to this world than the way we had learned to live, how to shun the type of living that kept us poor and lacking, through renewing of our minds daily, and that evil does exist. He showed us that there is a greater experience of community everyone can share with each other, leading to an enriched experience living on earth. We can actually experience Heaven here, too, if we believe in Him and follow these principles to better health and overall well-being. Jesus came to show us how to regain power—personal power and a gratitude that will elevate us to a higher frame of mind when depression threatens to take control, and how to develop a confidence that would face all the PITS you encounter, PITS of any kind that can never have room to flourish again. Made in God's image, we are all created uniquely whole—even twins each have their own individual DNA.

Jesus' message was very strong while He was on earth and still stands strong today. And the people of that time crucified Him, but the most exciting thing happened: He is the only man in history who died but is still alive! He rose from the dead and did that to show us that there is more to life than we can see naturally or will ever see physically, and He was willing to go the distance to show us this in His words written in the oldest book of the world and to share the knowledge of a supernatural world that is parallel to this natural world called earth. I once heard a preacher on television put it in these simple terms that I would never forget: He said that when we were born into this world, we were born into two standing systems that existed, whether we believed it or not. We either grow to live from God's economy/system or the devil's economy/system, or else as we grow, the decisions and choices we make tend to lead us on either road. One economy is invisible; the other is visible. He then asked which one we wanted to choose to live from. I have since grown to understand that for me, in God's economy it has been abundant, never-ending supply in every area of my life, and this can only be understood from the supernatural perspective. The devil's economy consists of the visible systems of this world, mainly the banking systems, educational systems, emotional systems, and more, and he was said to be very good at controlling even your pocket book and your ideas about yourself because of this.

I decided I wanted the never-ending economy, the one I can dream of having and actually have, that would never run out. Personal power, strength, healing, wholeness, self-control, abundance, and more is available to us in this supernatural economy. Who wouldn't choose this system anyway? But I didn't know how to get plugged into such a system. I also didn't realize that choosing this new undertaking was going to drastically change how I thought and how I perceived things. I was now going to change my whole outlook on life. I had to start from the very beginning of first understanding who I was and what were the benefits of claiming my new image that I was really created in and from. I felt strange, almost foolish, to believe in something or someone I could never see.

Yet, in God's image I was made. In that image, everything is good and perfect and forever youthful. No lack, no diseases, no shortcomings, no PITS of Health! So, why was my life so out of sync with the good book's idea of this great image that I was supposed to be operating from? Why didn't my parents ever teach me this knowledge, especially if it was meant for everyone who was ever born into this life? I had so many questions that caused even more confusion in my mind. All I knew is that I wanted to now live from this life. The life I had lived up until then had been very painful, confusing, cruel, and unkind.

If I was to make this change, it meant that I would have to give up everything I knew up to this point, but where could I start? If there was a better way to live without the pain and suffering, I needed it and I needed it now. I thought of how foolish it would look if I were ever to try and explain this to anyone, especially to a professional. After all, most professionals were successful and there was no higher force involved in how they got to be successful—we did it ourselves, by studying hard, writing the exams, and if we failed, we studied harder and tried again. We did it all ourselves. No reasoning mind could ever come up with a Savior who made us to flourish in all things good and only created us to serve Him and to tell others about Him as we become supernaturally successful. No one would ever believe this. No one can comprehend a God who is always working alongside our free will, to bring us to a point of wholeness, all because He made us, cares very deeply about what happens to us, and has developed this plan for us since before we were born.

When Darwin's theory was found to be flawed because it could not even explain the simple things of creation, people still chose to believe in his ideas. Why can we not simply choose to believe the words written in the oldest book existing on Planet Earth that even the best scientists are now relying on for answers to age-old questions that have never been solved, not even by the smartest scholars of all time? We can reason ourselves out of the very truth that stares us in the face only because we choose what we are willing to accept or not.

So we continue the debilitating journey in life, living from old and new comparisons—comparisons handed down through traditions, grandma's bill of rights that may have worked in the past, and hearsays of intellectuals who once lived. I remember when I first graduated as a Registered Nurse and did my pre-graduate studies on a surgical unit that I hoped I would eventually get hired on and become the greatest nurse who ever lived. My preceptor was a gracious little lady; she was highly skilled and taught me with much patience. I still remember she would praise me for every time I took the initiative and stepped out and performed within the constraints of the education I had received. On this unit were many skilled nurses who perfected every day and in every way what they did, and they were the best at it. They were a proud team of nurses. I remember showing up toward the last few days of pre-grad and vowing to be even better than the nurse who claimed she was the best on the unit. The only problem I had, and I came to recognize it quite fast, was that I was having trouble in the rotations that required me to do night shifts. I was nauseous in the mornings, I couldn't sleep when I got home, and I'd show up tired just to complete these night rotations. The still small voice of reasoning would say to me when I arrived on the unit: *You will never amount to anything except be like this pathetic group of nurses who think they are all that and then some...you can't even get through a night shift without feeling sick and you want to be the greatest nurse who ever lived?* I remember saying to myself, *the best, eh...in your dreams, baby.*

I still remember when I got hired full-time. I had been working for at least a few months into my career on the surgical unit. I wanted to quit even before I started, and at times I thought the other nurses picked up on this, so they gave me the most difficult patients to contend with. I remember saying under my breath, *Oh they will never amount to anything more than this job*. I had this attitude because they isolated and bullied me many times, and I also remember going home and crying out to a God I couldn't see. I would ask for Him to help me get through this, but notice I didn't compare myself to anyone in these moments. I just wanted the strength to get through the ordeal. I also realized it was easy to become exhausted just trying to keep up with improving my skills, and trying to find opportunities to succeed professionally. I was very determined to succeed at my profession, so through the subtle comparisons of skill sets, clinical abilities, and opportunities that were influencing this environment, I started to focus on developing my skills. If I was going to be the best-skilled nurse I wanted to be, I did not have to compare myself to any other students or nurse on the unit or in the hospital. But if I wanted to be better as an individual, I should be comparing the real self I sometimes displayed and the hidden self I was hiding every day. I also had to make an effort to focus on thoughts that I could use to help rewire the negative thought patterns that I had embedded within me and to start creating new grooves in the neurological pathways that would cause changes to occur in my health. More importantly, I needed to make the kind of changes that would affect the different areas of my life through the old and negative processing of my thinking mind.

Are you exhausted trying to keep up with a title, with an idea, or even comparing yourself to others who you think might be better than you? It was in a moment of total surrendering, not being able to keep up with the comparisons to others, that I made the decision to step into this so-called God's everlasting supply of all things He had for me, so I didn't have to get stuck living from the line of lack, the road of false comparisons and of failing demands. I wanted more. I wanted what no one else had. I wanted what I couldn't see. I now wanted what was mine, but how would I get it? I had to start at the very beginning. This beginning for me was more than just the starting point of a new life, new thoughts, and new attitudes that would change my life forever. I was determined to prove to myself that where I wanted to go and would end up was not based on where everyone else was or would go, but to undertake a path that could be much better with God and that I could also share with others.

Next, I recognized that if I did nothing about my situation, I would self-destruct and if I kept following everyone else, I would end up in ruins. I needed to make a new reference point to begin from and to be able to measure growth—personal growth—not a starting point of comparisons from the blind leading the blind to see who would come out on top as the better nurse. It was in these moments of being honest with myself that I felt in my heart that the only viewpoint that mattered was mine and in that moment of making this decision, it put *me* at the source of true empowerment, but at the same time I was one hundred percent responsible for what would happen next.

Professional leader, it is in the ownership of this moment that everything changes, revelations happen, irreversible healing transpires, and truth enters into the mind and heart and transformation begins. My core values were overthrown. What had happened? I realized that in my own self I was nothing. The dominant thoughts that had ruled my life up to that point were founded in this world's system and could only lead to negative victories and delusional thinking that couldn't even give life to anything, much less to the abilities I was seeking. It takes the same amount of energy to fail and to compare ourselves to others as it does to succeed and become a true leader with natural and supernatural abilities. The difference is that one will have no true power, while the other will keep empowering.

Out of nothing something started happening. I was now trend-spotting my behaviors and my actions. I was determined to change. At this point in my life, everything I thought I knew was thrown out the window. I wanted to know how to keep this positive change happening. I was greedy for more. I had gone to church every week up to this point, but now it was different. That weekend at church, the pastor said, "Some of us come week after week and hear the words of God, but never do anything with them." He stated that if we accepted God into our hearts, our minds would change and God would be able to enter into our lives, thus transforming our very being "right at that time... right now." I had heard so many messages from so many preachers week after week, but I realized I had known nothing. I had never asked God into my heart; how could I do this?

How can God live in anyone's heart...how would He do it? Then I discovered the scriptures, John 8:31-32 NKJV, "Then Jesus said to those Jews who believed Him, 'if you abide in My word, you are My disciples indeed. And you shall know the truth, and the truth shall make you free.'" I questioned this. Then I read further in John 14:6, Jesus said to him, "I am the way, the truth, and the life. No one comes to the Father except through Me." Also John 15:16-19, "You did not choose Me, but I chose you and appointed you that you should go and bear fruit, and that your fruit should remain, that whatever you ask the Father in My name he may give you. These things I command you, that you love one another. If the world hates you, you know that it hated Me before it hated you. If you were of the world, the world would love its own. Yet because you are not of the world, but I chose you out of the world, therefore the world hates you." Wow! This was a lot to swallow. What amazing words! It now made perfect sense to me what the preacher on television had been referring to when he said we were born into two worlds, and that we basically choose each and every day which we want to live by.

Up to this point, my life had been nothing but hurt, pain, emotional turmoil, and lack, even though I looked like I prospered and was very happy. I wanted out of this so-called physical world, out of the devil's system, and I wanted the system out of my pocketbook. Up until now, I had had really bad relationships, had not got along with some of the nicest persons because of suspicion, and had been stuck in a comparison zone that controlled my thinking about who I was, who I wanted to become, and who I could develop into. Enough of this system—I needed to make this change and it needed to happen now!

I still remember after working on the surgical unit for about a year, after a night shift, the nurse manager had come to me and said, "You will be a great nurse, but you need to start by not guessing at the doctor's orders...you transcribed the Gravol orders incorrectly; never let it happen again." I stood in dismay as she showed me the transcription orders that were sent to the pharmacy. "The doctor's handwriting was not very clear and the order looked like it read 25 mg Gravol po/iv before each meal. It actually was 50 mg of Gravol po/iv before each meal. No guessing games; call the doctor and always verify the orders." I remember going from feelings of *yes, I have conquered the world of nursing and I can do anything* to feelings of smallness and *how could I have made a mistake like this?* I was just starting out as a surgical nurse. What would this mean to my career, to me as an individual, if I didn't practice the patience of clarifying a simple order such as Gravol? I went home convinced that God needed to do something for me at that very moment or I couldn't survive nursing—not if I was playing guessing games with people's medication orders. Even though the manager had assured me that she believed I would never let this sort of thing happen again, I was not very sure of myself. Again, everything I thought I knew was just thrown out of the window. I couldn't compare myself anymore. I remember going home and crying in my bathroom to God, asking how I could have done such a thing. I asked if He would do what he said He would do and help me. I felt like I was about to lose control of myself; I was suffering inside as it seemed my old foundations were being tested, and I felt as though everything I had ever known that was based on my old perceptions had been shattered. I truly didn't know where to turn. I told Jesus that I had read in the Bible that He said all I had to do was ask. I was asking Him at that moment to save me from my own pain, from following others, the world, and to rewrite my life, as I had everything but was still so very empty. I cried so hard, I cried myself to sleep and had a great sleep after that. In the end, it was the first and the last time in my whole nursing career that I would ever make a medication error or mess up on any transcription orders I had received.

What I didn't know was that God was already working in me to bring about a positive expectancy so that everyone who was in my presence or who knew me would realize it one day. Once you ask God for something, because He is so good, He must provide it. If it was in His will for what He planned for my life when He created me, and for choosing to renew my mind so that the world's system would no longer influence my thinking, I was going to get it. At one point, I got stuck telling Him He needed to come into my heart and He needed to do it now! I didn't realize He had already done so the very first time I asked and had started me on a road to mastering the very fundamental keys to controlling my thoughts, negative behaviors, and actions that once controlled my very being and even my outlook on life. But, you see, it was at the point of confusion, death to the worldly ideas, beliefs, and actions that when I came to this final place of total surrender and helplessness, it carried more value than had ever been present in my life or mind at any given time since my birth because it involved bridging my physical self with my spiritual self, closing any gaps that were open to allow the negative and dysfunctional aspects of life to flow in and influencing my overall functioning.

Everyone must come to this place at some point and time in life. At that point, those who would have earned great power and wealth according to God, became poor in spirit. I feel this experiencing of falling from a position of good health, great power or wealth and having to face a crisis is what makes us become aware of the greater aspects of life, when we have to face ourselves, and rationalizing won't bring peace and we just cannot run away; there is nowhere to hide. There are no exceptions if we are to come to the end of ourselves for God to take over. The vastness of God's love for us is impossible to comprehend with our human, intellectual, or thinking mind. God has done so much for us that we are not aware of. When I surrendered to Him fully, that was the beginning of a total acceptance of me, with a new starting point in lesson 101 of depreciation of self.

This must occur for any deep appreciation to bud even while living in the depths of the PITS or in excruciating circumstances. Our appreciation for life will first be superficial until we put a strong emphasis on ownership for the real meaning of our own life involving these principles at work and the challenges we have come through with the help of God and our faith. Then we have testimonies, news articles, books, and other transformational materials that are widely available to us for helping ourselves and the society in which we live. But thanksgiving for what God has done for each of us to bring us through just because He loves us can be a real challenge. We don't feel as if we are qualified to accept this love and abundance to live a balanced life. He will equip us with a knowing and will lead and direct us to actions far beyond our means, and transfer the supernatural into our lives, developing a constant and renewing principle that transforms life, my life...your life. Then the *aha* syndrome kicks in and you realize that you were created uniquely, with no comparisons to any other person or thing, even if you were not physically or mentally or even spiritually aware of it.

Did you ever notice that when you went through something—as similar as it might have been to another person's experience, it was still very unique to you? Even in the PITS of Health, each of our experiences will always appear and be uniquely our experience. So let's change this area in our personal thinking and make our unique experience a positive experience with a new and solid foundation. We each have the ability to become uniquely perfect, and writing this book has taught me that this applies to me as well.

Many of the thoughts and ideas presented in these pages might seem familiar to you, but have been experienced differently by you and will bring about a change in your perception according to how you experienced them and what you have learned from someone else's experience. Even though we all will experience the same things, each experience will remain uniquely different in many ways that will explain our traits and other factors that build up our personalities. Other areas related to our perception of life, as well as other challenges we may have faced in the past, will become clearer to our minds once we apply any specifically learned or new principles. These learning curves become even more personally unique as they pertain to each individual level of application or experience.

You are extraordinarily formed in your genetic makeup and uniquely framed in structure of personal growth and possession of skills. We were created that way on purpose. Our uniqueness allows us to make a specific contribution to the lives of others, our work life experience, and the community life experience. You need to embrace this; science can even quantify this fact, for there are just no comparisons between each of us and what we bring to the quality of life and the overall environment around us. Even our footprints are individually unique! No competitions, no comparisons—it's just not necessary and it's simply that easy! You are unique and nothing can ever compare!

CHAPTER 5

Getting Out— Balancing Health and Life

Let's for a moment consider the unique functions of the liver. The liver is a very large dark-red gland that is located in the right upper portion of the abdomen and just beneath the diaphragm. It has many functions that include storage and protective functions. For instance, it is a storage and filtration system for the blood, it secretes bile, converts sugars into glycogen, breaks down fats and will store them temporarily as fatty acids, and helps regulate blood volume. In many more functions, the liver builds up essential proteins and stores up certain necessary vitamins until they are needed by other organs in the body. It disposes of worn-out blood cells by sending them to the kidneys for disposal through the urine. It destroys bacteria and will detoxify drugs, alcohol, and environmental poisons. It balances the sex hormones and will police the proteins passing through the digestive system. The liver will even reject and neutralize acids and will send them to the kidneys as waste.[3] These are just a few of its functions—the liver is a very important organ to the body. It is basically the police force of the body for balancing health. There are other very important and vital organs apart from the liver, but the liver is the main organ that works together with the other organs to make sure that the body is balanced.

But there are things that can hamper this extraordinary organ and its proper functions. Most of us can become out of balance in many areas of our lives, and this can cause serious consequences in other areas. When we are not fully balanced in

---

[3] Saunders – *Encyclopedia and Dictionary of Medicine, Nursing, and Allied Health* – Miller & Keane 4th Edition

health, we can suffer from depression, lack of energy, and many more diseases, creating imbalances that in turn will disrupt every area of our lives. Again, looking at the liver as an example, when liver function is impaired, dysfunctions or disorders may be created. To mention a few, the liver can become damaged by disorders and by diseases such as hepatitis, an abscess, cysts, tumors, uncontrolled bleeding, obstruction in its day-to-day functions, and more.

Likewise, when we are weighed down with doubts, fears, unhealthy behaviors, lack of sleep, insecurities and more, we are shifted out of balance and sometimes, because we are focused on work, money, and comparisons to others, we miss noticing the processes functioning behind the scenes that are building up our thoughts and ideas. Sometimes it takes a great disappointment, a death, an accident, disease, or extreme pain to bring past PITS to light. Sometimes this discovery comes much too late. Other times, we are privileged to get a glimpse of it before it evolves into something much bigger and deeper. Like the liver, which polices the body and creates a balance working in conjunction with the other organs, we need to step up to the plate at the end of the day to start this process. But sometimes, when our life is too busy or in disarray, our thoughts and minds are everywhere else and we have no way of seeing that we are heading for a big pit until it's too late.

Balancing health and life will take a bit of effort, especially if many other areas we are about to identify are also not in accordance with good health. None of us will be one hundred percent perfect, but we can still make changes that will be beneficial to creating balance for a good life. We tend to think that nutrition is the only key to great health. What about sleep, meditation, regular relaxation periods, and exercise? Do you skip meals for a smoke? Do you spend time drinking alcohol to help you relax or sleep, but never find the time to relax and unwind naturally, without stimulants, for example by meditating? How much sleep do you really get at night? Have you ever tried meditating on God's goodness even in the smallest of things by just sitting there and thinking about them instead of worrying profusely about the problems that have become your priorities? Is your diet consisting of fatty foods, sugars, and high amounts of salt or refined carbohydrates? These are all practices that will throw you out of balance and change your life forever and most of all put you in a dysfunctional disposition, leading you to the PITS of Health.

Diseases, dysfunctional habits and dysfunctional thinking go hand in hand, forming the PITS. If we are to be balanced and healthy for a better life, we must take *full* responsibility. We cannot leave it to chance that things will work themselves out, or because we have compared ourselves to someone else who is just like we are, and so we continue to strive this way. You really don't know what road will lead to the PITS they will have to contend with, but one thing is for sure, they will be taking you along with them. The question is, how important is your life to you? How long would you like to live in this beautiful world? Regardless of the hurts and pain you have or have not experienced, there is a better way to live. I am not promising you the moon, but I do know small changes bring big results. Again, it's a matter of choice, your personal and unique way of choosing.

I once asked a professional if he exercised. He replied that his job kept him so busy that he had no time to take breaks. He stated that he was so busy at work that it was like exercising, and to come home and do more exercise or to join a gym would be insane. Yet, he was severely stressed out and could not tell me how he planned to stay healthy. He did complain that he had high blood pressure and pains in his legs and hands at times. I asked him when was the last time he had had a doctor's appointment for a physical or even lab work to police his health for better control of his body, emotions, and balance. Most professionals believe the old saying, "If it ain't broke, don't fix it." This belief will send you down the path to PITS of Health that, if left undiscovered and unchanged, will have serious consequences.

The end result will be a short, miserable life and heavy medical bills in the years that you should be enjoying life. What will you choose today? Become a serious partner to your health and your life and experience the goodness that was intended for you at your birth. Meditating or spending quiet times with ourselves can help to bring clarity and insight into the PITS that keep us captive in bad practices, leading to imbalance and ill health. Change is easier than we think, but to remain in a destructive state of living is really easy too. It may be hard work to turn around with our own efforts, but the good news is, it's never too late to try.

There are many great programs, books, classes, and teachers in the market who have wonderful materials geared to creating a good and healthy meal or to teaching how to balance work, activities, exercise, and issues of mental health and more. In this book, I aim to give you an overview of areas we face in life that affect our health and well-being, causing deterioration in our ability to function, which happens when we are not fully balanced. I also aim to help you stay focused on areas of necessity for longevity in good health and to help steer you out of destructive holding patterns that are formed in our minds from our experiences as we grow from childhood to adulthood and into our lives as professionals and leaders. I further aim to provide insights to a better alternative. Most of all, I would like to raise your awareness to what areas need absolute attention immediately if you are to avoid the PITS waiting to trap you in ill health, disease, and mental obstruction. If it ain't broke, it's a great time to look at what may need fixing in the distance, and all of us have something we would like to change, shake loose, or address in other ways before it gets out of control.

Again, go back to the previous chapters and to your personal lists and identify areas where change is absolutely necessary. Even areas that look good right now can have the potential to be changed for the worst. Revisit them and make notes of things that could cause an imbalance for you later on in life. If there are many areas to change, you may want to seek out a professional who has the expertise to help you in that specific area. If you pray for change, it may help to take some practical action to go along with your prayers. Be smart and seek the correct help as needed. If you do nothing, you will self-destruct and if you continue to follow others, you will most likely end up in ruins.

CHAPTER 6

Spirituality on Purpose

God has a habit of picking up nobodies and making them somebodies – MyBible.com

This was one of the hardest chapters for me to write, mostly because so many people believe in so many different things—different gods. Even believers in God will falter, have doubts, and be filled with despair when instead, as believers, we are called to be an example. While it's true that no one is perfect except for God, we still have a responsibility to show others how to live worry-free, doubt-free, and filled with faith. If we are inefficient in our service to God and to others, we tend to perceive and deal with our problems by blaming them on an external situation or influence, or we may ascribe them to coincidences. People who are curious about who God is will turn away because of how we display these inefficiencies in our own lives. This makes us no different than the person seeking a new way to live and is just another form of comparison. Some people are looking for examples and will use other people's lives and challenges to measure where they perceive themselves to be, thus achieving a better view of themselves from other people's misfortune. But none of us can be as perfect as God.

Our inefficiencies even put a negative and restrictive aura on how we expect things to turn out or even on our health expectancy for life which, in turn, affects our day-to-day thinking, even inhibiting God's work in our lives. Yet He still loves us with an everlasting love and pushes past our resistance to open us up to fully receiving what He has to offer us—a full life supernaturally charged with success in all areas that is free from stress, sickness, and disease!

Whether you are a Christian or not or do not believe in anything or anyone at all, as mentioned in Chapter 2, it has been shown that everyone believes in something even if unconsciously, and will have a god of some kind in their life. Money, a job that we love, material wealth, houses, cars, a position—all of these can become a god. Once these objects consume our focus, they become priorities over everything else and are like gods that control our lives. This adds stress and pressure to our foundation and weakens our resistance to disease, response to crisis, or the ability to bounce back after an accident or terrible loss.

Even though God the Father is never pleased with such actions, He is still always with us waiting for the opportunity to forgive us and to come into our hearts and lives to make a drastic change for us. And yes, this change is superior to anything we will ever have experienced or can imagine. He waits for our approval to have His help, to give us the strength we need to refocus our lives, and to begin to trust in an everlasting love that exceeds all imaginable love. Whatever we will need in life and for health He has already given us and is waiting for us to accept it.

At the fall that occurred at the beginning of time here on earth, the devil stole our rights to living happy, healthy, and wealthy lives when he tricked

Adam and Eve. He stole our birthright and became ruler of the earth. He keeps us captive by creating doubts about ourselves, God, and other positive things in our lives. He creates fear, insecurity, and most of all disbelief that God is real, and so we continue to operate without ever reaching our true and real potential. This applies even to the leader/professional who is on top of the world and thinks that they have made it there by their own means and efforts. This enemy can create this delusion easily in this world because he runs it—it is his system we live by. He causes you to become discouraged; he causes pain, hurt, and ill health. The madness that is overtaking us in the world today is created by the devil, yet we blame God because we have a lack of knowledge of who God really is and why He cares so much for us. God made this world before the devil devised the plan to steal it, and even today, with no hope left for many of us, God is still in control.

Jesus came down to this earth to show us there is a better life while we are here, and there is heaven when we are through living here. A good person does not automatically go to heaven when he dies just because he did well. There is a process that must take place, and we must be intentional about it.

Whether we are good people, great leaders, or whatever we think we are, we must believe that Jesus came to take us back to His presence away from the claws of the devil, and died a brutal death devised by the devil using people of that time. The devil did not win. There will be an end to this life and world. This is written in many places of the Bible, but one stood out for me in this context, in Acts 4: 12, "Nor is there salvation in any other, for there is no other name under the heaven given among men by which we must be saved."

We must seek God first and ask Jesus to forgive us for all the wrongs we have done, which includes dysfunctional thinking, and to come into our heart to live. That is the only way to experience freedom, full health, and true wealth. It's hard to imagine this, I'm sure—to give your life to Christ, a man you have never met and to a belief and faith found in the oldest book of the world that has divided many families and nations to this day. But it's the only process. Just as we can believe to get a promotion or get "lucky at winning the lottery," this is all blind faith—something we don't see as yet but believe it can be achieved. Once you have asked Jesus into your heart, everything about your life starts to renew itself and an ultimate process of change takes place. At the mention of the name of Jesus, the devil will have to leave you alone and everything about you starts to repair itself and bring you back to a whole state in body, mind, and spirit. Once you give your life to Christ, you become automatically His. You gain a new relationship and recreation through the son-ship and daughter-ship of God, and the supernatural takes over. 1 John 5:14-15 states, "Now this is the confidence that we have in Him, that if we ask anything according to His will, He hears us. And if we know He hears us, whatever we ask, we know that we have the petitions that we have asked of Him."

Folks, God made us and knows everything about us. He knows when you are lonely, in pain, or discouraged. He knows what you have done, what you will do, and what you are currently going through. It is no secret that He sits high in the universe looking down and has created each and every one of us. No matter what we have done and continue to do, He will always love us because He lovingly took the time to create us. It is the devil's tactics that keep us trapped and make us think we don't deserve the unconditional love that is offered so freely to us, all the time, with no restrictions or conditions. When God comes to live in you, He is greater than any living force and will help you to overcome loneliness, grief, pain, lack of self-control, depression, lack of resources—you name it, He can do it. He wants to see all of us, not just a few, change and transform to truly become His children!

While I was writing this book, I became very ill. At first I thought I was coming down with the flu. I had gone shopping with my best friend and upon returning home, I felt unusually tired. Aside from the usual daily pains that I have managed to live with, I thought it was nothing. Now in my knowledge of God, He never puts sickness on anyone, and it is not His will that we become ill. I already knew this. I knew that, according to scriptures, every day the devil has to ask God's permission to test us and if God allows it, it is for a reason where His glory can become evident in the midst of it all, also to strengthen our faith in *Him*. I went to bed that night, but realized I was becoming weak. I couldn't eat or get up even to use the bathroom. I was able to take sips of water and forced down some blueberries, knowing that I had to find some way to keep up with the nutritional aspects if I was going to get better. But I got progressively worse. I had a phone call from someone who did not believe in Christ—a dear friend who told me that was God punishing me. I knew that was not true and then she asked me how come I was so spiritual but suffered so much. I tried to explain in my weakness that it was the curse of this world where we are born into sin and the devil was the main player, but God is always faithful and will always be there for me, even if I can't physically see him.

Another friend, however, was very supportive. He came after work to take care of me and helped attend to my illness. After a few days of sickness, weakness, and weight loss, we spoke to my family doctor and we were told to get to the emergency department as soon as possible. At first, I prayed and asked God why He was allowing this on top of all that I had recently gone through and continued to go through. I told Him that He had promised me in His Word that I would receive anything I asked of Him that was good. God cannot lie and He honors His Word; I even reminded Him of that, too. I had asked God to see me through to the age of 95. The funny thing was that even though I shook my hands at Him, I felt a strange peace in myself, a kind of knowing that His presence was with me. I wasn't worried, but I wondered what it was that He thought I had to learn.

I started to ask His forgiveness if I had wronged anyone; all this took place on the way to the hospital. As we arrived at the hospital, even getting into the wheelchair was a big chore, and I never thought I would get through that moment. We arrived at the emergency department and I was triaged, and then the wait to be called to see the doctor was on. As I sat there in the full waiting room, it looked like we were going to be there forever. Then I heard a small voice in my mind saying, *well, I guess God left you to suffer here, didn't he? If they admit you, you are never coming out of this place alive—did you know there is an outbreak of C Difficile?* I did not become afraid, but spoke back: *Devil, I am rebuking you right now in the name of my Father, Jesus, because He is still with me and will keep me safe.* Then I heard again, *oh really?*

We were called in to see the doctor and my friend wheeled me to the room where there was a stretcher waiting. Lab work was done, an intravenous started, and a full history was taken. We had gone to the hospital where I had previously been employed, and I felt very comfortable knowing I was being cared for by the very colleagues I had worked with. Then the devil whispered again; this time the small voice said, *ah, they haven't seen you in awhile. Now everyone will know you have become a loser at home and are disabled, what will you do now?* At that moment, my feelings and emotions got in the way, and instead of keeping my eyes focused on the fact that God was with me every step of the way, I started to cry uncontrollably. I started fearing the worst. Was the accident finally catching up with me? Was I still trying to regain wellness by overdoing it? What if I didn't get out of here? What if I died? I had no will in place, my son was in Ottawa, and all kinds of thoughts entered my mind at that point.

I discussed with my best friend who was to be called if I was to die. What I forgot to do was pray. I was focusing on the worst instead of staying focused on the love of God for me as His child and that I would get through this. In that moment, I had totally forgotten all of God's promises for me that are found in His words, for each and everyone of us. God does not lie. He is a good God and wants the best for each and every one. He will never leave us where we are in life. I found myself forcing myself to pray. I prayed, Lord Jesus, I am afraid and I don't know what to pray; please help me, as you promised that if I ask you anything, I will receive it. I know sickness is not from you, so please help me to get

Spirituality on Purpose 111

through this; help me to know that you are here.

Before long, I fell asleep. It felt like it had been hours when the specialist came in and said, "Ms. Desmond, I have reviewed the results of the tests completed and I just have a few more questions for you." On the completion of the answers, he said, "If you did not come into the hospital when you did, it could have ended differently. This is a rare condition you have developed. It is called Rhabdomyolysis." Even as a nurse, I had never heard of such a diagnosis. I thought I was contagious. He explained that the condition occurs when damaged bones and muscles break down and shed into the bloodstream. "If you hadn't come into the hospital, your kidneys would have become clogged and failed and you would have died," the doctor added. I thanked God immediately that I had not remained in bed another couple of days and that we had taken my family doctor's advice to get to the hospital immediately, even if I thought it was probably nothing but a bad case of the flu. Then a peace came over me and a knowing arose inside of me that said, *I was with you and made sure you got here safe and you are in good hands, with familiar professionals you know, and you will be alright. I will never leave you. You are my child.*

I could feel the tears welling up inside of me. They were tears of gratitude.

I was transferred to the medical ward, where I stayed for several days. To explain how God's grace carried me through – the first room I was in I shared with another woman. During my bouts of nausea, I would pray: *God, my life is in your hands and I love you.* I started playing some of the sermons I had on my computer to build up my confidence in Jesus again, but my roommate rebutted. She didn't care to hear any of it, so she would turn up her television very loudly, so that she couldn't even hear the nurses speaking to her. Then there was an outbreak of C Difficile in the room, and this woman was affected. My colleagues moved me to another room. I remember the nurses telling me that if there would be any more outbreaks even here, there was no place else to go. In going through the ups and downs of the illness, I continued to surround myself with God's words and promises. Then I was placed into a room with a woman who had been there for about six months. Her son came in every day, sometimes twice a day, to see her. She was a Christian, but no one had addressed her spiritual needs. Her son was a non-believer, but enjoyed the sermons that I played every day, and so did she.

I noticed she had perked up when I played them and stopped crying at night. She didn't complain of pains at night anymore. I got to the point where I was playing the sermons more for her than for me. She was starting to speak to her visitors as if she was renewed. I now know that she had missed the spiritual side of herself and was glad to have some of it come back into her life. It was as if she had made peace with herself hearing the sermons.

Finally, I was discharged home with the admonition to take it easy, as I was not totally out of the woods as yet. The cardiac enzymes were still very high, but home was the safest place for me to be, due to the outbreak in the hospital. A week after I arrived home and was recovering slowly and with much care, the woman's son called me at home. He told me that his mother had passed and that he wanted to thank me for playing the sermons. He said that he was not a believer, but his mother had been, and she had not had the spiritual aspects of her life looked after. No one in the family was a practicing believer. I assured him that she had gone on to be with the Lord because she had been able to come to grips with her spiritual self and that was what she had missed and was now at peace. Then it dawned on me that in the midst of my trials, God was blessing me and using me at the same time. I had to have been there for this woman; she needed what I had to offer. It was God using my situation that the devil had meant for harm, to bring good to both of our lives. Had I not been in the hospital, the outcome would have been totally different, but through my being there, we both had our spiritual needs met, even though we were not aware of it. I was in awe at the way God turned everything around for the good for the people who loved Him. I laughed at the devil; I said to him, *You tried to take me out with a rare condition? How stupid of you to think you can outwit God!*

While I was at home recovering, I had a flashback of an experience of my encounter with Jesus. It was the day He came to me or I went to Him. I think this flashback was meant to seal my faith in Him that my life was in His hands. I had totally forgotten about it. When I was 21 years old, a very dark moment came into my life. I was told by my doctor at the time that I had to have major surgery for the damage that had occurred inside of me from the brutal rape. I was to have my fallopian tubes removed and a possible hysterectomy. I was told I would never have children, due to the severe damage I had suffered. It was not what a 21-year-old woman who had already gone through so much was hoping to hear. I contacted my family to let them know I was going into the hospital. My grandmother, who was the most disciplined and faithfully devoted person to God I knew at the time, prayed for me over the phone. I still remember walking up the long hill to the hospital in a blistering winter storm and being admitted. I felt I was the loneliest and most unloved person ever. I had lived on my own since I was sixteen, had a lot of friends but could not find anyone who was close enough to talk and to cry with, or to whom I could even admit I was feeling very scared.

The day of the surgery, I was prepped, and as I drifted off, the nurse came and told me that my mom had called to say she would not be able to arrive before the surgery. It was the worst snow storm ever, and my parents were coming from the west end of town, but the nurse assured me that my mother was going to be there before I would wake up. This thought did not offer much comfort to me because I had a very strained relationship with my mother. Then the doctor came in and asked if I was ready. He said it was to be a substantial surgery lasting several hours and he was going to try to do his best for me. I still remember just wanting to die—the loneliness, hurt, pain, and feeling of being unloved—it was just unbearable. Even now, writing these words still brings a tear to my eyes. They had given me the prep to induce sleep, then I was wheeled into the operating room. Back then, this was the process. I remember distinctly as I drifted off to sleep crying my heart out and wishing I could die, I came into the whitest and brightest light I had ever seen. I felt warm and comfortable there. I remember asking if I was dreaming and Jesus came to me and called me His child. He told me He loved me and what I was feeling would pass and that He would not let anything happen to me. I asked if I was in the operating room. Then He hugged me and told me He would be there, too.

I remembered feeling so loved and filled with comfort. What I didn't realize was that I was in the arms of Christ Himself. The next thing I remembered, I was awakened and asked if I was alright by the doctor who had done the surgery. He was an African doctor, and all I could see were his big fat fingers and later was told by my family that I said, "Wow, look at your hands, your fingers are so big and fat!" It became a joke as the story was told over and over throughout the years. I remembered the encounter with Jesus, but was afraid to talk about

Spirituality on Purpose 117

it because I didn't want to look like I was crazy. I did eventually tell my grandmother, and she said it was Jesus who had blessed me and that I had been special from birth. I asked if I was so special, then why did all these things keep happening to me?

This is the trick of the enemy to keep life so busy in all the different areas that are important to us, so we can forget the really important thing that should matter to us in life instead, and that is our relationship with God. You see, we cannot keep holding on to the broken pieces of our lives; there is going to be pain and hurts, but we cannot use them as an excuse to stay the way we are, either. Changes can take place if we let them. Proud people are very insecure people. Inferiority frees us to a prison of our past, past failures, anxiousness, depression, anger, guilt, and guess what—it will seep into the holding patterns of our health, creating PITS of Health!

Yet even in our darkest hours and moments that no one knows of, God is there! This is more than an attitude to help us resolve these things or areas in our lives. It is a dependency, a dependency on the most powerful person who ever lived and still lives! The enemy, or the king of this world, is your worst foe and is a liar, and just in case you didn't know, he has been defeated! His defeat took place when Jesus Christ died for everyone, and yes, He did that all for you and for me.

I watch many faith-based programs on television to help build up my spiritual health and to keep me focused on God. I had accepted Jesus as my Savior when I was twelve while I attended the Emmanuel Temple Seventh-Day Adventist Church in Buffalo, New York. In our teenage years, my sister and I spent all our summer vacations there with relatives. I grew up in the Adventist faith. It was the denomination that my grandmother felt, back then, was the closest to the Messianic Jews, a faith she had adhered to all of her life. She lived with us, and both of these faiths were influencing my life, but I was still experiencing some emptiness inside. Something was missing from my spiritual life and I didn't know what it was. In my adult years, my faith was strengthened as I watched many of these faith programs for three years every morning, crying immensely. I think it was in year two after the car accident had occurred. I had missed nursing and my friends at work, and it was being in so much pain every day from the accident and having to attend so many doctors' appointments that broke me. One morning, I was so fed up and started yelling in a very loud voice, "Lord, why me?" Then, as I turned on the television, I saw Joyce Meyer, a television evangelist, come on, and she started talking about her own life—being raped by her very own father every day of her life until she was in her late teen years. I was in shock to see that she was a happy person and was able to speak so freely of what had happened to her. It was as if God had sent her to the television to speak directly to me. I wondered how she could admit these things on national television. I heard Joyce say that she had had a devastating start, but she was going to have a successful finish, and the tears just streamed down my face. I realized that my pain was bad, but there is always someone else who has it worse than we do. I cried for hours. I was surrounding myself with spiritual programs and attended weekly church services, but none had a more empowering effect on my life and changed my outlook more than Joyce Meyer did that day. I thank God each day for Christian television, for the incredibly encouraging programs that I can attend at the church, and for being able to read inspiring books to help build up my spiritual health and life. These were what I desperately needed to regain my focus and rebuild my faith. Together, these programs and activities supported my well-being and laid the foundation for healing to take place in many areas of my life. I couldn't wait to get home from the horrendous appointments so I could feel the comfort of God's words penetrating my life through these various aspects, closing the gap slowly on the emptiness I felt.

You see, I believe that because I chose to take the first step by deciding in my attitude that I was desperate for change, God started making a way. I was too caught up in feeling sorry for myself and God knew it. He knew that what I needed was far better than any medicine I could have taken at any time. Sometimes when we are at the breaking point and become lost within ourselves, He already has a permanent fix ready for us, but we must reach out in some way to get it. Even if words can't express it, just merely say, "Jesus, help me," and He will be there swinging into action. His love is more than we will ever need—I now understand this. What do you need from Him right now in your life to fix your PITS? Just ask!

The more we make a conscious effort to change the destructive behaviors that we recognize, the more God is able to do a great work in us transforming our mind, transforming our lives. Once you decide to stand with God, you become an heir to His Kingdom and to all the good He has waiting for you, and the devil then has zero power over you because God will place a protective hedge around you. No matter what you face after this, God will see you through and help you to be faithful as well as strong to do it. A true revelation of God brings a resolution in your life, against the people who have hurt you, in your health and in your circumstances, for with God "all things are possible to those who believe." He is ready to revolutionize your health and to put you on a path to positive change. Why wait until tragedy hits your life to go searching for God? When we don't have His power in our lives, our homes fall apart, our marriages fail, we have stressful jobs, ill health controls us, and we are led to the PITS of no return. Then it all shows up in our health by way of disease, a condition, a mental problem or issue, and this keeps the cycle going, and going and going to no avail.

Everyone has a purpose to be born and to live a great life, even if you don't know what it is at this present time. But sadly, not all of us will discover this before we die. The force of faith is a very powerful force. Just as we have strong desires for material wealth and happiness and they manifest themselves into our lives, the same principle holds true for the desirable things of heaven, and when we embark on them earnestly, the very PITS of Health that once held us in captivity will begin to disappear through the medicine and healing that are found in His words, and we will again experience peace of mind, comfort, strength, positive expectations, and outcomes in all areas of living. I once heard someone say, "Everyone is a believer; they just don't know it as yet." We can teach each other to live free of the burdens that cause ill health, disease, and pain. You can start manifesting your potential when you know who you are. Remember, just as decisions decide your wealth, decisions decide your health, too. It was Zig Ziglar who stated, "When things aren't adding up in your life, start subtracting."

Religion holds you captive with laws and worldly dos and don'ts, but a true relationship with God will transform you and will revolutionize your mind; then God's interceding actions work on our behalf and will transcend all that you are facing at this present time. You can have successful friendships, a satisfying job, great health, a growing business, a bestselling book, and even become a legend, but nothing brings more success than having a sincere relationship with God, and He can do above and beyond anything we ask or desire. He will put His seal on you as a sign of ownership and protection. I dare you to try and see what happens.

God's words are *medicine* for the soul! So use it liberally!

CHAPTER 7

How to Develop Your Personal Tracker

Tracking your success will take perseverance, but it can be achieved if you really spend time developing this area of your life. If you have been diligently following the exercises in the previous chapters, then you have all the information you will need to complete this task. By now, you will have identified all the areas of change that are necessary. Whether it is a personal hurt, mental pain such as depression, or a physical condition that is plaguing you, it can be dealt with. The idea of this chapter is to get you on a path that will help you identify the areas that need to be changed immediately, areas that will require some time to change, and areas where you will need help to make change happen deliberately. But at the end of this chapter, you will be able to put yourself in a position to not only track your success, but to keep track of the things that once held you captive, whether in thinking, spoken words, or health, and to stay on top of them so that you become aware of them and that they can never creep up and take over you or your life again.

In your journals where you have identified what has led you to be tossed into the PITS of Health, you would also have identified the dysfunctional things or the dysfunctional attitudes, behaviors, and circumstances that led you to this area of your life and have kept you there—the strongholds, so to speak, that would have taken much of your time and several days to accomplish in that exercise. Kudos to you because I know that identifying certain things would have brought back to mind memories of the challenges that created the pain and suffering, but on the bright side, this will now not have power over you, since you have discovered that there is a much better way, especially after reading Chapter 6. This new way of thinking and the ability to change are yours right now! This is a very important exercise because you want to now point out the recurring themes, experiences, and conditions that were prevalent from the last exercise and to now list them on a new page. Beside each one, list the change you want to make. This is very powerful. It's like rewriting your life. Make sure it is stated in positive words, almost like making an affirmation. Words have power and bring to life the good, bad, or unjustified, so make sure you are setting yourself up for a successful progressive change in your personal tracker of your body, mind, and spirit. So, to clarify, on this new page the title is "My Personal Tracker."

In the column to the left of the page, put the negative disposition you had identified from the Dysfunctional list that must change, and on the right side of the page, put a positive outcome that is simple to track—a positive decision to overcome whatever that negative is. Be good to yourself.

For example: *depression, no self-esteem (rape, loneliness, hurt, etc.)* ... "I have decided to forgive and to put behind me any thoughts, feelings, and people whose actions remind me of this pain every day and in every way. I will affirm today that I have always been beautiful and I vow to look for and to find the beauty inside of me each and every day starting now. I am created in the perfect image of God and past circumstances can never change this. I am very beautiful indeed!" (Or, for a man reading this book, "I am very handsome indeed!")

Another example: *pain (disease, health conditions, mental anguish, etc.)* ... "Jesus died to make me whole and healing is mine; it is mine to accept, and I accept this healing now. I am healed from internal mental anguish that controls my focus."

Now these are just a few simple examples, but you must claim the positive and most superior outcome that will defeat the negative that has been controlling you up until now by adding an action that you can do, but please make it as positive as you can. You can make it as simple or as complex as you wish, but the bottom line is to have some sort of action that you can be responsible for. When we accept our share of the responsibility, we create ownership, and with ownership come results. It's like creating a new script for your life, as stated above, and you have a right to choose what goes into your script. Someone else choosing for you means there will be no personal engagement, therefore any real attachment invoking change will also be absent. No one else can do this for you; it is your life, you must do it!

These are just vague examples, but it is important that you make it as real or transparent and meaningful to you as possible. It is what will help you to take hold of the PITS that are disturbing your health, the very things that weaken your immunity or cause the rut you are currently stuck in. But creating a foundation for change will transform your outlook in those same areas and strengthen your desire for the specific change you need to make and to make it stick for lasting results.

Don't rush through this exercise; take the time that you need. For some of you, your list will be very long, as much has happened to you. But it's important that you persevere. For me, it was hard to get through just the first item on my list because it evoked pain every time I tried to list even the dysfunctional part revolving around trust issues that I was responsible for, so it took me a while, but it can be done and you can become a new person with a brand-new outlook on an old pain or hurt.

Leaders are the absolute worst at this; we put on a persona as if we were invincible and, as previously stated, we drown our own issues into someone else's pain. If you have asked Jesus to come into your life through reading this book, then ask Him to help you through your list and possible pride and He will help, especially in the difficult areas! This is what I had to do. I then found myself kneeling on the floor, crying out asking God to forgive the gang of men that brutally raped me, and now the incident is only in my memory bank and cannot hurt me anymore, even when I think of it. Now I find myself talking about it to help others, just as Joyce Meyer was preaching that very morning. I had to face my worst fears, but God brings you through it all for an excellent and dynamic finish.

Once you have done this, seek out the positive words or the opposite of what you have experienced—words that will help keep you on track and diminish feelings that will keep you bound so that you can stand steadfast and not stray again, or that would help to keep you from the culprits that would bring back certain feelings of fear, hurt, and despair. Make a note of them, look them up in the dictionary, and pick out the very opposite to the negative ideas, words, or feelings and put the positive outcome of that negative situation into another positive sentence that describes what you want for yourself. This is a great practice with many benefits to consciously help you put the PITS in their place.

I know this exercise involves a lot of work, but it is well worth it. It will no doubt not be an easy task because all that we have experienced will have a strong hold, especially on our emotions. It has been buried there for as long as we can remember. For every negative experience, there is a negative word; for every negative word, there is a positive experience or positive word waiting to be manifested into your life—now seek it and find it and make it part *of who you want to become from this day forth*. No, this is not wishful thinking, but it sets a new foundation in your mind to work with. God was and is able yesterday, today, and tomorrow to help you start anew.

You can choose what you want to let into your life. Why not practice by choosing the positive outcomes instead of remaining a victim or remaining under the control of an old experience that is gone? We are the ones who keep the old occurrences fresh and current. Now it is time to get rid of them and to change the slate, but it has to start with you and will take supreme effort. You can read dozens of books and they all will have ideas, exercises, and much more on how to change a thing, a condition, or belief, but the bottom line is that it all begins with *you and GOD*! Ironically, some people like to stay in the PITS that bring them to ill health and keep them powerless, because it feels safe, comfortable, less challenging, and takes no personal effort at all. What about you?

Unfortunately, some of the changes you make may require you to drop some people in your circle who have been sucking the positive energy out of you, directly or indirectly, perhaps by keeping your past hurts and pains in front of you and by reminding you daily about them. You might have to change a job, give up a position, or stop going to some places you have been going just to receive a false sense of comfort, and these are part of the discoveries we must make if we are to become very successful going forward. This process creates a new outlook after the pain is placed into proper perspective, and even if we can't change a diagnosis immediately, for instance, this process can and will induce a better outcome or outlook in our mind, guaranteed! Your thought life will change and a new self-esteem will begin to emerge. You must be honest with yourself. You have to make an effort to track the things that hold you back. It will not be easy. You MUST persevere. This will also help to strengthen your immune system and prepare you for the change that is about to take place in your life. It's time, it's your time. Remember there will never be a perfect way to start, nor a perfect time to finish cleaning up areas in our lives where change is necessary, regardless of where we are in life! So just do it, make that effort to change now. Make the effort to take control of your life now!

CHAPTER 8

Principles 1 – 10

Principle #1:
Meditate

- Meditation is very important because it frees the mind, releases stress, and releases feelings of negativity and insecurity.

- It helps pain subside and it makes you appear lighter and stronger.

- Meditation connects you to your greater self that is found within you, and to God.

- It brings clarity of mind and the Holy Spirit speaks within the silence of your being.

- It refocuses your desires and helps you to forget about your negative self.

- You become more appreciative of yourself and of your surroundings.

- Meditation has many health benefits.

Principle #2: Develop a Great Attitude

- Having a great attitude develops a positive outlook on life.

- It keeps your moods up.

- It allows you to beat negative circumstances much easier and you are able to better face any calamities with a positive outlook.

- It allows you to see the good in any situation.

- It fosters good health, improves bad health, and is a perfect conductor for healing.

- A positive attitude creates opportunities in areas where we have failed in the past and opens unexpected doors for advancement, especially related to work.

- By having a positive attitude, you attract good in all things and attract great people into your circle of life.

- It helps you to always see the bright side of things, and everything will always look good to you.

Principle #3:
Maintain Healthy Behaviors

- Healthy behaviors help to establish grounds for total health and increase healing in every area of life. They set the foundation for a good life.

- Adequate sleep allows the body to unwind

and release stress and fatigue, thereby relaxing the body and creating cellular renewal.

- Get lots of fresh air and sunshine; they stimulate the purification processes of the lungs and many other body functions.

- A well-balanced diet built around vegetables, fruits, grains, and nuts, along with drinking plenty of water, helps feed the body with the proper nutrients to build healthy nerves, bones, cells, and endurance. It builds up immunity and deters any form of disease. It's important to have breakfast, as it prepares the brain to function after it has rested while you slept. Supper should be light so it is easily digested. Heavier meals should be ingested early in the day so there is enough time for them to be adequately digested.

- Rest and relaxation are even more important if you work long hours regularly. They also help to alleviate stressful attitudes and behaviors that are taxing your body and can impair your thinking while harboring stress within the body systems, such as your muscular systems, and more.

- Exercise is vitally important to keep the acids secreting out of your body that are held within the joints, such as the knees, elbows, and hips. Regular exercise keeps the body from experiencing muscle fatigue while building strength within the bones. It also allows you to sleep better at night, is great for relieving stress, and helps to keep the flexibility of your muscles and joints. It relieves pain, increases libido, improves moods, and much more.

Principle #4:
Surround Yourself with Good People

- This is equally important because people tend to think they know what is good for us, so if we surround ourselves with good people who have great attitudes, they will help to foster good behaviors, attitudes, and outcomes.

- They will feed your spirit with positive thoughts and ideas because it is what they expect you to do for them as well.

- Good people are positive people; they lead exciting lives, are healthy, and will not tolerate any negative input into their lives.

- They are supportive without tearing you down or holding your past against you.

- They will always look out for your best interests and help you to appreciate the good things in life.

- Positive people are very outgoing and really don't have any time to dwell on negative ideas, thoughts, attitudes, and beliefs.

- They are your best cheerleaders in times of distress.

- They can help boost your self-esteem and inner strength.

- They are action-oriented.

Principle #5: Weight Control

- Maintaining a healthy weight keeps the mind and body fit to be active.

- Helps to keep you alert and aware.

- Wards off systemic diseases and prevents conditions typically linked with obesity.

- Helps to alleviate pain and suffering within the body.

- Keeps the joints free from added stresses and weight-related conditions.

- Gives longevity and life to body and mind.

- Proper weight control helps us to rebound faster from any unforeseen challenges.

Principle #6: Self-Talk

- Monitor your words; they give life to your soul.

- The way you speak about yourself can build you up or break you down.

- Incorporate positive words into your day; it will change your day dramatically.

- Positive self-talk promotes your mood in a good way.

- If you engage in negative self-talk, you will attract negative people who are feeling the same way.

- If you engage in positive self-talk, people will want to surround you and build you up.

- Positive self-talk helps to keep a positive attitude, regardless of what you are currently experiencing, and to offer a great outlook on life.

- Positive self-talk will heal a negative self-image.

- Monitoring self-talk will lead you to a place of positive acceptance among peers.

- Your positive self-talk becomes contagious to those who are around you daily.

- Positive self-talk helps us to be more compassionate toward ourselves and others.

- Negative self-talk creates negative changes within the brain and body.

- Negative self-talk can encourage PITS of Health and keep us in the ditch of despair.

- Positive self-talk heals the mind, body, and soul!

Principle #7: Reflection

- Reflection is great as it helps to bring clarity and focus to the current moment. It promotes a positive mood, as well as rest, sleep, and peace of mind.

- Reflection answers any intimate questions we may have hidden inside ourselves.

- Reflection can help to eliminate stresses as it leads us to the next steps we will need to take to achieve our goals.

- Reflecting on past negative situations keeps you looking back and you become a hostage to your past hurts, conditions, and pains, so be sure to keep your reflection looking forward.

- Reflection lessens hurts and takes the power out of emotional pain.

- It keeps us in proper perspective about a matter or thing.

- It always helps to move us forward, especially when we are stuck.

- Reflection can give us power to conquer any negative holds on our life.

- Reflection can enhance or take away worries; again, it depends on how we view ourselves.

- Walking enhances reflection and brings clarity to mind issues.

- Reflection allows you to exercise gratitude in the small things about yourself; being grateful in life goes a long way.

- Be aware that too much reflection can also keep the mind excessively busy—so aim for keeping balance in all things!

Principle #8:
Ditching the Negative

- Ditching the negative takes a lot of effort, but will bring great results if you persevere.

- Ditching the negative means ditching negative friends and family, too, which can help to eliminate a lot of the stresses in your life.

- It's not easy, but gets easier the more you practice ditching.

- It's relieving of the old self, as much of what has happened to us will have been negative.

- Ditching the negative can automatically prompt change if we seek the good in every negative situation. Negative people will keep looking at the negative in you, while positive people will notice a positive change in you.

- It immediately brings a new insight to handling any situation and offers a new perspective.

- Ditching negative attitudes and beliefs realigns your thoughts, actions, and deeds.

- It keeps you motivated and makes you more accepting of yourself and others.

- You create a better aura, as negativity keeps a dark, gloomy aura around you.

- It frees you from inferiority and a substandard position.

- It creates a breakthrough in health and other conditions.

- It makes you look healthy and even wealthy in your appearance.

- Laugh! Faking a laugh will induce the real thing, and laughing releases negativity from the body. It also promotes a positive feeling of well-being.

- It improves self-talk, promotes successful relationships, and a positive outlook on life!

Principle #9: Giving

- Giving to a special need allows you to reflect on your own needs.

- It helps you to validate your own position in life.

- It creates a sense of self-worth through giving of your time, efforts, energy, or a thing.

- Giving promotes compassion, which in turn builds us up.

- It keeps you open to receiving—we have heard that the more you give, the more you get.

- Finding simple ways to give benefits our mood, mind, and positively impacts health.

- Helps us to forget about ourselves.

- It keeps us humble if we do it out of the goodness of our hearts.

- Giving brings a true perspective to our real needs, wants, and desires.

- It exposes our true character and capabilities.

Principle #10: Community

- Being involved in the community, even in simple ways, helps us to develop better coping practices as we see how others cope.

- It helps to adjust the thinking we bury inside ourselves that creates malfunction in most areas of our lives.

- We become more aware of what is available to us.

- It helps to bring us out of a rut and promotes our capacity to love others just as they are.

- It keeps us connected to the important things in life.

- We can realize from being involved in the community that we need to make important changes in our lives.

- It opens us up to positive people who can assist us in making much change.

- It keeps us current in our thinking and approach to problem solving.

- It improves moods, attitudes, and deters stresses, even if it is only for a moment.

- It encourages reflection on personal issues we desire to change.

- Being involved in the community exposes who we are as a person, leader, or professional.

- Although these principles are randomly selected, there are other areas not covered that are equally important to seek out in order to help you improve your circumstance, health, and other areas of need. These are just a few that were selected to help develop a sense of awareness of the vast areas of our lives that could land us in a pit of ill health, but you may wish to extend these as you read through them. What other areas are necessary for you to focus on for your growth and well-being?

CHAPTER 9

Reaching Out, Setting a New Foundation

Transforming our minds will take many steps if we are to be successful. It means being willing to fail over and over again until we master the mind's eye and our old way of thinking, but it can be done. Perseverance is the key to helping us to keep focus if we are going to create a new foundation in our lives and will eventually dismantle the PITS that lead us to ill thinking, negative practices, and deteriorating health. Transformation can be achieved!

You must be transformed physically, emotionally, and spiritually, loving yourself, as this is where the enemy speaks to us and keeps us looking back to a place we no longer want to be. Everyone craves to be loved the most. Self-talk in a positive way will bring the unique breakthrough regardless of what is going on around us. The mind is a powerful instrument that can be retrained no matter where we are in our lives. Power often comes to a leader or professional if they keep up practice and self-control. The same is true in changing any area of our lives, be it health, a circumstance, or position. It can be done—not overnight, but every effort ultimately leads us a step closer to our new goal.

You will remember that the exercises in Chapters 7 and 8 offer suggestions on how to make a new plan to help you move forward. For every negative, there is also a positive, but you must take hold of this thought first in your mind, then the body will follow. Even if you are currently facing a horrible diagnosis, you must believe that change is possible. Regardless of how things currently look physically, there can be a positive spiritual change waiting to manifest itself. As in a theatrical play, many times we allow the curtains to come down on our lives instead of letting them go up to the opening of an exciting moment, and that exciting moment can come with self-empowerment and tenacity to change.

After receiving the diagnosis of the rare condition of Rhabdomyolysis and experiencing body pains every single day, not to mention terrible headaches, I wanted to give up on my life. I had never thought of suicide before, but I started entertaining thoughts of an easy way out of this misfortune I was placed in. Although I knew it wasn't my fault, nevertheless it was what I was experiencing. I was sent to a rehabilitation specialist to see what she could do to help direct some form of therapeutic engagement that might assist my family doctor going forward. The day of the appointment, I remember sitting in her office waiting to be called, and all kinds of thoughts starting to enter my mind once again. I tried to shrug them off by thinking that maybe she was exactly what I needed, she might give my doctor ideas on how to assist me to get through the day with less pain, control the headaches, and perhaps conquer this new diagnosis I would not accept. I had been practicing every positive affirmation I could about myself before the visit, regardless of how I was feeling.

You see, if you have a plan for the old thoughts, imaginations, and attitudes, when they creep up, you can choose to see the positive side. But if you are struggling to find anything positive and it is not easily located, you will have to make something up on the spot, or defeating thoughts will come and take over. Realizing this, a fight began in my mind as I was determined to remain open-minded to what this specialist had to say. As it turned out, the visit was positive and helpful beyond what I had expected. It is important to remain open and positive, but we often tend to fall back to a familiar pattern of thinking or reasoning instead of pressing on and pressing through to a better state of mind. If we are to lay down a new foundation within our thinking mind and emotions, we must deliberately walk over the old and familiar, and we must do this over and over and over until we can see victory even in the smallest of ways. When the mind gets it, the body will most times automatically follow.

Go to the mirror and take a long look at yourself. Start at the top of your head by admiring your hair—the texture, the color, and the flow of strands. Move slowly to your face. Look at your eyes as if to inspect them—the color, the contours, and so on. Look at the rest of the face, moving to the neck, shoulders, and the rest of the body. Embrace yourself, the unique beauty or handsomeness of who you are. Even if you are a twin, you will be uniquely different from the other. In your unique state, realize there is only one of you. So embrace yourself, even hug yourself. Make a vow today that from now on you will seriously make every effort to look after yourself. A vow to eat properly, to think right about yourself, to sleep properly, giving yourself enough hours so the body can unwind and rest. Vow to exchange the negative things in your life for the greater things and possibilities to come. Remember instead of having the curtains come down on your life, vow to have them go up. This is the start to laying a new foundation to life and to health.

If you are having difficulty just getting started in any area, reach out to someone you trust whom you see in a positive light and ask them to help you get started. You will have to tell them what you are doing, and this is a good thing as it makes you responsible to get the support you need, and it holds you accountable because now someone is aware. Don't be surprised if that individual wants to join you on the journey to self-renewal; this is what often happens. In building a new foundation, you must choose to look up, choose to have good health; choose to have a good outlook on life regardless of what comes your way. You must choose not to be oppressed. You must be selfish and put on the positive hat and right thoughts about you. You cannot give up! You must force yourself to set this foundation based on the changes you are willing to make and not based on what you currently see; what you are seeing physically is the old plans that, if left in place, will keep bringing you backward. Trust the Supernatural God to step in and to work for you.

If you should slip backward in thinking, forgive yourself and keep moving on. To help build you up, write out some positive affirmations that are meaningful to you and say them every day. These words can come from inspirational books or even the Bible. Set a schedule to help you do this exercise. It is intended to help rewire your thoughts to where you want to go deliberately. The opposite of faith is fear, and if you are not faithful in doing this, you will become fearful of not being able to pull off the changes you need to make and will start to second-guess yourself. Remember, in laying new foundations, you must treat yourself with love and respect. The past is now behind you and the future has been waiting a long time to embrace you with benefits beyond measure.

Rewiring your thoughts will bring you to another platform and yet another platform and yet another until your perspective changes, and this will ultimately be the new foundation you have worked hard to achieve. Here is where you will be starting again. It will be enlightening, new, and exciting, and only you can step forward and take hold of the NEW YOU! It starts with one step at a time, one moment at a time. With every step, you will develop a new outlook; every move forward moves the PITS backward and further away from you, and you will begin to wonder why you did not do this before. The changes that were made will become much clearer to you, and people will start to notice them in you. You should develop the perspective of living with positive expectancy!

Your mind is a steering wheel. The direction in which you turn your wheel, the body will follow. Hug yourself daily; this helps to confirm with the body that the mind is pleased with the new you. Usually anything you wish to change starts in the head first, then the body will always follow. Please remember this. This is the one true concept you need to reinforce to help you build a new foundation and lay down solid ground work for change: for change to occur, you must renew your mind. When you renew your mind, everything around you will begin to transform!

You need to know what you want for yourself. The exercises in the previous chapters should have introduced a vast variety of areas for change. Put your efforts into what will work best for you. If you plant oranges, you cannot expect apples to grow. Oranges are what will grow. The same with renewing your mind—you must be forceful in developing a healthy mind regardless of what the body is doing. Be clear about the positive outcome. Search for what you already possess inside that is valuable and positive and build on this. That will set the stage for a permanent change to take place and will build a very strong foundation indeed.

The next step is to view yourself in a higher light of what you used to see yourself in. Do this with your health and other areas. When someone asks how you are, express yourself from these new heights with value and love. Again, if you are finding yourself facing some difficulty, reach out to someone you know who can help you or just refer to this book and use it as your pep talk to yourself. Remember, once you achieve it in your mind, then the body will follow. Change your attitude about yourself, and your mind and heart will love you with persistence. Even if you are living with a disease or condition, this will also change how you view yourself with that disease and you will no longer be defeated by these circumstances. You can now be in control instead of the condition controlling you. I am not suggesting this is easy to do, but it is very possible and can be done. You must challenge your insights of the disease, of yourself, and of how you see your future self if you are going to be successful and in order to maintain control on your new platform, your new foundation. Try to build or cultivate a new set of instincts to help guide your decisions and feeling or emotions in the future. Persevere; you are now on good ground.

Whatever you need to help you build your new foundation you already have; you just need to find it inside of you, but you must keep digging past the old trash that needed to be cleared away so long ago, and as you keep digging, I guarantee you will find it. But don't let fear make the decisions for you and keep you from turning this new leaf for yourself. Please also don't view your changes or outcomes according to your feelings. The grass may always appear greener on the other side even if it isn't, but it's the change in your perception that makes it appear so.

I just made a statement that I will repeat again, but this time I will provide proof. "Whatever you need to help you succeed at anything, regardless of how complex life may be, is already inside of you." This includes seeds of greatness or seeds of depression. What we sow we reap. Everything you need to move forward and to create a new foundation has been placed inside of you from your birth. We lose that awareness as we grow and go through life battling hardships in general, and just a few people will ever regain this truth in life. The same power God used to raise Christ from death He has given to us. God lives in us and so does this power. Ephesians 1:19-20 states it very clearly, "[19] and what is the exceeding greatness of His power toward us who believe, according to the working of His mighty power [20] which He worked in Christ when He raised Him from the dead and seated Him at His right hand in the heavenly places," (NKJV) and so we know that this same power He has placed in us. We therefore have as much power as we are willing to exercise over our lives. The work has already been done for us.

CHAPTER 10

Practice What You Preach

Now that you have successfully laid down a new and valuable foundation for moving forward to deter any new PITS of Health, you must practice what you preach. As mentioned in Chapter 9, if you plant oranges in your garden, you will not expect apples to grow. The same is true for embracing your new image. You must watch your words and self-talk. You cannot expect your foundation to grow strong if you don't stand up for the changes you desire or have already made. If you want change, you must keep practicing to see change. You can't expect to see change if you state, "Yeah, but... I don't know what will happen; I thought I wanted this, but..." You have just negated the positive outcome you worked so hard to achieve. You must practice what you preach. If you have made a certain change, for example, if you no longer drink coffee and eat meat, but now you are out socializing with friends, you cannot say, "Oh, I'll have one cup of coffee and eat two hamburgers, just for tonight." Even if your friends say to you, "Oh, it's just one night; it's not going to make a difference." Yes, it will make a difference. You are now negating all that your mind has put in place for your body to follow. Then, a day later, the attempts to discourage yourself will surface because you did not practice what you have been preaching to yourself. If this does happen, forgive yourself and move forward.

You must be steadfast in your journey and not be easily swayed in the simple changes. This will make you more successful with the difficult changes. As time goes by, you will become much stronger in your decision-making process, but you must maintain your foundation in order to come out on top. That is why you must decide beforehand the changes that are necessary, the changes that are priority, and the changes that are just entertainment. The mind knows the difference, but the body cannot differentiate and like a robot will follow what the mind tells it to do.

In the state that I'm currently in, as I have previously mentioned, I experience body pains that are unbearable. There are times when I can do nothing but lie in bed after taking pain medications, and as much as I never want to feel defeated when my body speaks, the mind will still yield to the body's promptings. But I refuse to have these physical pains conquer me. I still managed to get this book on its way, even though it took some time; I still manage to tell others of what I have learned that can help to better their health just by simple conversations, for instance in store lineups, and I am still able to put into practice what I am telling you. What I am saying here is that my mind is beyond what my body tells it, and I, too, am practicing to call this great power forth, but the power can only be strong and successful in our lives if we hold fast to the faith and believe. I believe there is no doubt about that; I just need to remain faithful in what I say. I celebrate the small victories, forgive myself when I accept defeat on a very painful day, and hug myself instead of always feeling sorry for myself or beating myself up.

On a day that I feel well, I treat myself to a manicure or pedicure, or I may visit the lake and celebrate nature, forgetting all about the days that I'm not able, for whatever reason, to function normally. So I am also aware that the journey is a task that requires endurance. Would this mean I will ever give up? No, God forbid, but I am able to share this insight with you. We as professionals or leaders are strong in positions, but often succumb in personal trials. I would like to see that change and all of us become strong all around and support each other, which is why this book is motivating me also. I had a lot of time for venturing into the spiritual realm to know that better things do exist, but many of us do not have the time or inclination to do so. So, I have done some of the work for all of us. Am I a Bible freak? To some, I might be, but I have no shame in saying that if I had not discovered what I am writing about, I would be lost and my life would have remained a total mess. I have grown in ways that help me to control how I feel even while suffering, and I find relief just knowing that God gave us the ability to master the things that the devil keeps sending our way to try and stop us from living a life free of pain and suffering. Hence, I am able to still create a new foundation in my health by starting with the small tasks until I can master the big things that are trying to hold me back; and you can, too!

Remember, to lay a new foundation, sometimes it is necessary to reach out. I reached out to the oldest instruction book, the Bible, for knowledge, comfort, and peace, but this is only one means of reaching out. Then, the change of anything must start in the mind before your body can follow. Another example is getting out of debt. You want to get out of debt, so you think of ways to do so, and then once you devise a plan, you start to do the things that will lead you to getting out of debt. If you want to obtain a degree at school, you will think of what you desire, get registered, and start taking courses. Before long, you will graduate and have a degree. The same is true for overcoming the PITS of Health that keep most of us captive. To help me in my own journey, I have an affirmation that I say that goes something like this, "God's goodness and mercy will follow me all the days of my life, and I will live to be a healthy 95-year-old." What affirmations are you writing in your mind, heart, and body for laying out your new foundation and to practice what you are preaching, especially to yourself? This is going to be a very important question to keep in mind moving forward.

I once saw a quote that said, "The most important decisions are not to be made with the mind; they are to be made with the heart. So when you have an important decision to make, check in with how you feel, not how you think." (author unknown)

CHAPTER 11

Perseverance—A Determining Factor for Longevity

"Take care of your thoughts when you are alone and take care of your words when you are with people."
~ Melchor Lim, Inspiring & Positive Quotes

You are probably familiar with the term, "stick to your guns." To have longevity in anything, you cannot be changing with every tide that rolls in and out of your life. If you have been reading this book and diligently applied many of the exercises, thoughts, and ideas, you will have instated a new and strong foundation that is flexible only to positive advancements. It would offer a new start to the new you as a leader or professional and place you in a new perspective for improved health. You would have had to push past some of the old familiar thinking and health practices and to be able to beat the odds in other areas of your life. Kudos, as this is never easy, not even for the strong at heart.

However, in order to have a foundation that will be built to last, you have to keep pushing forward. The quote presented at the beginning of this chapter speaks volumes. When we are left alone, our thoughts can really play a number on us. I have explained several times why this happens. When we are with others, they can be very persuasive, especially if it appears that they have it all together. This is a trick stemming from our perception of how things appear to us. Yes, the grass may look greener on the other side until you get there and realize it is not so. The same is true with perceiving people to be well balanced and having no flaws or issues. They, too, would have had a struggle or two in order to try and maintain their balance, and their fight will never be the same as yours, no matter how much you may have in common.

You must guard your mind and your words that you speak about yourself, whether it is over a health issue or any other condition. Remember words bring to life the things we speak, and the things we speak often fester first in our thoughts well before they are given life.

Longevity is determined by what we put in place for long-term use. This will even include the affirmations for rewiring your mind, soul, and body.

If you plan to bake chicken for dinner and place it in the oven, then receive a phone call from a friend and end up talking for more than an hour, chances are you are going to let the chicken burn to a crisp. The same is true in hoping for longevity. If we just make weak and shallow changes to get by, how long will they last? Can they stand up to future challenges you may encounter? What plans do you have in place for an unexpected turn of events? Are they plans that can only strengthen your foundational choices or will they crash and break your foundation down again?

The same is true for your health. Have you made a revised health program so that you will have the opportunity to change the conditions in your life, control diseases, etc.? Will that plan you are living with only get better or will it deteriorate over time? Will your new health plan land you in the PITS of Health once again? Check the new plans you have made and reflect on them for strength and longevity, not just for how good they appear from the outside or on paper, but also what your heart is directing you to do from the inside. Life has many turns that can test the strength of the strongest tower, especially over time. But if it is built to last, no disaster can ever tear it down again. Thus, it can stand up to the test of time, and this also applies to the new thoughts or perceptions that we now have developed about ourselves. If they can be easily broken and if there is no room for positive, flexible advancement, then there will be no longevity for them.

Longevity for any plan that is in place is like putting on an armory that must be sturdy so that nothing can knock it out of place. It cannot rock the new foundation and will stand up to anything. Fortunately, I can say I have found such armory and longevity in the promises that God has placed in each of us and in the Bible, that good old instructive book. It is a solid rock and equips us to proceed, thus leading to a successful victory so that nothing can defeat us, whether in mind, body, or spirit. Healing may be slow, but it is sure. What will you equip yourself with today to keep you mentally healthy so that the body can follow? Find it, test it, and then apply it!

CHAPTER 12

Success Indicators

A successful indication to change simply means you are now *connected, corrected, protected, and perfected*! **This means you are renewed.** Say this to yourself out loud: "When it comes to my health, I am connected, corrected, protected, and perfected in Jesus Christ! I claim these words in my life today." These are powerful words that should be repeated several times per day until they seep into your spiritual self, your mind, and finally your body.

What you are telling yourself is that you have confidently made the necessary changes in moving forward that will protect you from any unforeseen slipups and you have built a strong foundation that only you and God can change. That is a very strong revelation to affirm and to develop a strong hold in.

In the previous chapter, you would have put your longevity plan to the test; now, working with the concepts offered in this final chapter, you are sure to become very successful and the PITS of Health will not prevail in your life any longer. Living with a health issue will no longer control you, but you will now be controlling it even if you are living with pain daily! You have been built with this power to be successful, happy, and healthy, and in stepping forward through this new way of life, you can continue to develop positive strongholds for yourself until you become totally whole and balanced again!

The last phase to the plan is to develop and put in place indicators for flexibility and resilience that will promote your plan, no matter what comes your way in the future. With faith, you are stretched from the inside, and a well of determination will always rise up and will flow out of you; this also will affect others. You become a reservoir of good resources and blessings for yourself and to share with those around you, over and over again. You might ask how it could be possible to be positive all the time. Yes, it is through your new perception of things. You can choose to have a positive outlook regardless of whether you see immediate or physical changes or not. Life, including health, is a personal choice; so is staying positive regardless of what happens. Be happy and grateful for the small changes; they will fuel the bigger changes.

A friend of mine recently told me a story about a woman who was born into a family that suffered extensive poverty. At the age of 6, she had to assist her mother in making a living for her family after her father died. At age 12, she quit school to work full time. She only knew to clean, and so she did this for many years to help her mother and her other siblings. When she was 18 years old, she got married and within six months of marriage got pregnant with twins. The twins were stillborn, and so she fell into depression. About three months following the stillbirth of the twins, she fell in her bathroom and became unconscious, was admitted into the hospital, and was in a coma for two years. During those years, her husband divorced her, and her mother was now taking care of her. After two years, she came out of her coma and had to have both her legs amputated for gangrene. She made it through this surgery, but developed a heart condition. She still lives with this today. She greets everyone she meets with a big smile. Hearing of her story, many often feel pity for her and think of her misfortunes as a curse in life. After everything she has gone through, she stated that she was happy to be alive and happy to still have her arms. She has never once viewed her life as a curse but stated that God was still in control of her life and had big plans for her. What a courageous statement this is! Many of us have never experienced anything close to what this exceptional woman endured. We crumble at the simple things and at worst hate ourselves, even mistreat ourselves, for the so-called misfortune in our life.

This woman has developed a highly successful indicator that is fail-proof, and it is communicated through her hearty smile that she shares with anyone she encounters. Her breakthrough from the PITS of Health keeps advancing to greater success indicators because she has learned to master the pitfalls; they have not mastered her. Her willpower also is flexible and foolproof, so she is always able to move forward positively. She has what I would term "forward, flexible thinking." Her body has been afflicted, but her spirit is unbreakable!

Although this story is an extreme example of overcoming and persevering, we all have the same drives in each of us. I included this story because this book can only address a few principles to fighting and overcoming the PITS, as this is a very big subject. But what is mentioned can get our engines started with the first steps to ownership and renewal.

Zig Ziglar stated, "Success isn't just about what you accomplish in your life, it's about what you inspire others to do." If this final phase is difficult for you to put in place, consider this: I had to do an assignment once that entailed looking up my name and gleaning all positive attributes about my name, so I did. I searched the Internet for the meaning of my name, Jennifer. Some of the results I received said, *Jennifer was fair and smooth, was King Arthur's Queen. Jennifer is passionate, compassionate, intuitive, romantic, magnetic, a humanitarian, broadminded, and generous.* There was more, but I stayed with these explanations that were inspiring in explaining who I was through my name. If there was anything listed that appeared negative, I would find the opposite that was positive to write down. After all I have been through, I am determined to live with peace of mind and pray daily that this peace permeates my body even while I am in pain. I took this list and made an affirmation for each one, or a wish list, if you prefer. I said it every morning and sometimes at night for over three months.

One day, I had a phone call from a friend I hadn't heard from in a very long time, and throughout the conversation, she tried to tell me I was closed-minded because I didn't want to hear her whine as she had done in the past. Some people tend to be stuck in a rut, but after many years of no contact, I expected her to have changed. I didn't make any comments to any of her requests or offer any advice, either. Remember, in this chapter, we are discussing "successful indicators." When she insisted I tell her why I did not comment and offer advice, as I had done in the past, I found myself telling her that I was very generous to sit for twenty minutes to hear her whine about something very simple while I was experiencing body pains and that I was showing compassion in doing so, as I no longer entertain negative people, but because I had not heard from her for a very long time, I was exercising a humanitarian spirit. She became very upset and told me I was full of myself and hung up on me. It was an indication to me that I had been successful in transforming certain negative behaviors and habits I had once had. This incident really allowed me to see how I had grown and to measure the strength I had placed firmly in my new foundation.

Mental health is always the number one factor in our health paradigms that suffers the most and is always subjected to attacks. It always holds the key that will alter the cellular functions starting with our bodies, but we must guard our thoughts and our words to make sure they fit the image of wholeness we continue to seek. When you can fully achieve it in your mind, your body will also be able to fully achieve it physically. I have made a good plan for recovery by affirming these principles for myself, too. In this case, my plan was mostly made from the list of wishes or affirmations I had made from my name that were positive.

You have much to say about your destiny, and you are always in a position to reclaim it, too; no one can ever change this unless you allow them to. Work on strengthening your success indicators and you will be that strong tower that can stand against much and will never give up. Start by standing in faith, walking in faith, and living in faith. Get to know God and His plan for your life and believe you can achieve great success with a partnership with Him. This will lead you and you will achieve the greatest changes you can ever make for your health.

"Only one who continually reexamines himself and corrects his faults will grow."
~*The Hagakure*

Remarkable and revolutionary success is ahead for you in reclaiming your health today. All the best to you in your healthy and prosperous living! All the best to a NEW YOU!

About the Author

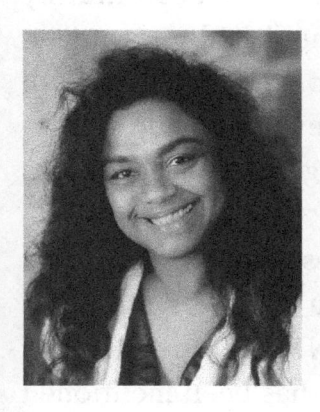

Jennifer Desmond resides in Oakville, Ontario, Canada, and is the Founder and President of a nonprofit organization called RROPE – Rexdale Rebuild Outreach Programs & Education. The organization serves many women and is an advocacy for the marginalized populations in the Rexdale, Ontario, community. Jennifer is a nursing professional with many years of achievement in hospital and community settings. She is very resourceful, organized, and is a strong patient advocate. She is passionate about nursing and uses a creative approach to the promotion of health and wellness within the community and in the nursing profession.

Jennifer worked as a full-time Surgical Nurse for over 10 years and was a preceptor for many nursing students. She has worked as a Cardiac Exercise Supervisor in the public health sector, in Hepatitis B Immunization Clinics at schools, as a volunteer practitioner of humanitarian services, and more. In November 2008, she spearheaded a successful health symposium as a community initiative supported by local municipal government. She is a Nursing Ambassador for "Team up with Nursing Campaign" who developed and implemented impact-driven nursing career presentations to large audiences of Grades 7 through 9 students, promoting the nursing profession.

Jennifer was awarded the World Organization of Natural Medicine (WONM) 2009—Merit of Achievement. Ms. Desmond has been mentioned in numerous publications and received a "Leaders in Learning" Nursing Award & Scholarship from Ryerson University in 2011 for Outstanding Community Volunteer Nurse. Most recently, Jennifer was the recipient of the Mt. Olive Seventh-Day Adventist Church Community Service Award – 2014, for her organization's dedication and support in donating to the food bank over the last several years.

She served in leadership as a Faith Community Nurse and as a Health and Stewardship Director for her congregation, planning holistic programs with her team, and delegating responsibilities in order to serve the large church congregation. Jennifer developed and presented wellness presentations to community organizations, including many churches, retreats, and schools, to promote health and well-being. She holds a solid track record in leadership, public speaking, and program development. Jennifer believes that if we empower individual families to develop a healthier lifestyle, this will create a better outcome for the determinants of health affecting the children in these families, which can have a major impact on the future of our society.

Jennifer Desmond is currently compiling a workbook with exercises to accompany this book. Please visit our website for updates on the publication date, or to join our mailing list:

www.overcomingthepitsofhealth.com